WHO'S BEEN PEEPING IN MY BED?

WHO'S BEEN PEEPING IN MY BED?

Barbara Moss

Who's Been Peeping In My Bed?
Barbara Moss

Published by Aspect Design 2009
Malvern, Worcestershire, United Kingdom.

Designed and Printed by Aspect Design
89 Newtown Road, Malvern, Worcs. WR14 1AN
United Kingdom
Tel: 01684 561567
E-mail: books@aspect-design.net
www.aspect-design.net

Cover Design © Aspect Design 2009
Original photograph © Alastair Miller

ISBN 978-1-905795-35-2

Contents

This is devoted to my loving family,
Mark, Jevan and Aidan and, of course, my loving Mum.
Dad always remains in our thoughts.

In writing this, I give my appreciative thanks to all
the doctors and nurses who have cared for me, the wonderful
St. Richard's Hospice in Worcester and Bowel Cancer UK
who have helped me at every stage of the way.

'Faith is taking the first step even when you don't see the whole staircase.'

Martin Luther King

Foreword

Barbara has had a challenging emotional roller coaster to ride in the two years she has been part of St. Richard's Hospice. When you first meet her you might miss the steel at the centre and only notice the softly spoken, educated lady with the engaging smile. However, there most definitely is steel there and her contribution to a much needed change in government policy was clearly and forcefully presented.

Illness can sap strength and dampen enthusiasm – which makes it even more impressive when someone carries on being strong and enthusiastic about the business of living. Barbara has. She is creative (although she would add 'not talented') and shows no sign of changing her mind about the importance of living life creatively and well.

As a chaplain and given that I'm speaking about a Christian person, it feels right to quote Martin Luther King: "Faith is taking a first step when you can't see the staircase." If Barbara hasn't already got this as a motto, I think she should adopt it immediately.

David Knight
Chaplain, St. Richard's Hospice.

Introduction

Barbara Moss is an inspirational woman and I am delighted that through this wonderful book many more people will now be able to read about her brave and moving story.

It's been a real pleasure and a privilege getting to know Barbara and Mark over the last year or so, and I'm very glad that Bowel Cancer UK and our pro-bono lawyers have been able to help them in their campaign.

Combating cancer is a big enough battle for anyone, and it is unfair that so many people find themselves in the position Barbara and Mark did: having to fight bureaucracy as well as the disease and to make financial sacrifices to get the treatments that can help them.

Thankfully, more and more people are becoming aware of the inequities that patients face and Barbara's story has been at the heart of the very high profile debate surrounding this issue, including in the media.

We are hopeful that as a result of this greater awareness and because of positive stories like Barbara's, more will be done by the Government and others to make things better for patients and those who care for them. The charity will continue to do all we can to help make sure that this is the case.

I know that everyone at Bowel Cancer UK joins me in thanking Barbara and her family for their support and in wishing them all the very best, both in Barbara's continuing patient journey and with this life affirming book.

Ian Beaumont
Director of Communications, Bowel Cancer UK

Author's Note

In reading about my journey through cancer, please understand that I have written about my experiences as I have seen them; sometimes, things may appear to be different from reality, especially when undergoing trauma such as this. I have explained medical terms and conditions used in my treatment as I have understood them and accept that they may not be clinically correct. I have also changed the names of all medical staff but apart from this, my experiences are related as they happened.

Comments can be left at:- whosbeenpeeping.org.uk

1 *All the Trees were Green*

I've just noticed the catkins on the trees and it's only the fifteenth of January. The branches are still bare, but on every leaf notch stands a perfect droplet of dew that glistens in the morning sun and it reminds me of Christmas. How the time has come round again; another complete cycle.

If you're lucky, you enjoy your work, the family relations are generally good, the kids are friendly and one day leads to the next. This is as it was for me. It was really only in the summer of 2006 when certain things weren't quite right. Mark, my husband, and I were on holiday caravanning in Picardy and I was getting unusually tired. 'Oh well, I'm getting older,' I thought. 'Perhaps this is how it is when you're fifty-two'. Mark loves his guitar and I found myself taking a rest each afternoon while he sat outside playing. I would try to join him later and we would sing together. We had so much fun and I never thought any more of the tiredness.

A new school year started in September. I had put in a lot of preparation and was enthusiastic to see my classes enjoy their lessons. I was sharing a number of groups with a lovely lady, Justine, and she had made special files to record what we had covered each lesson. She was so methodical and that suited me just fine.

Before we knew it, half term was on us. Mark and I went to

Cirencester for a week, changing the campsite at the last minute as the booked club site was refusing people due to water-logged ground. We were very pleased with the location but I noticed myself getting a little out of breath walking up a slight slope that ran from the toilet block back to our pitch. 'I must start my exercises again,' I thought as I felt quite unfit to be panting so readily. I had been to the doctor's before going away as I had experienced stomach cramps and she had prescribed drugs for gastro enteritis. These had helped but the pains were still there and I thought that I would go back to see her before the end of the holiday. Once school started, it was always difficult to think about health and I didn't like taking time off; I hated the thought of other people taking my classes. I liked them too much!

On our return from Mayfield Park I started my exercises each day. Like before, I expected to build on what I was doing as time went on and get fitter but, instead of them getting easier, I was finding it harder to maintain the same amount, sometimes giving up. I did see the doctor and she thought I may have a hiatic hernia, gave me some stronger tablets and referred me to a consultant at Evesham for an endoscopy. This is a minute camera that is pushed down your throat to see what is really going on inside. The whole thought of this I found revolting but I was lucky to get an appointment after my day's work on a Monday. To my dismay, I found that the consultant was off sick and the hospital was unable to contact me. I had to rebook my appointment for Thursday but this time I had to take time off from school.

I got to the hospital in good time for my eleven o'clock appointment and remember still waiting until half past two before seeing the doctor. She was a fantastic lady and, even though she was running late, spent an hour with me. I was so concerned for the patient who was still waiting to see her after me. I was given a chest x-ray, which was clear, and blood tests were taken. I had a hard raised area just below my chest and she was obviously very concerned about this. By now, I had been reading up about my symptoms on the internet. The word 'cancer' had been cropping up but I thought that this couldn't really be happening. When I asked her directly whether this was in her thoughts, she was sensitive but direct in her answer that it was a possibility but we would have to wait for further tests.

My drive home felt endless; I was having to concentrate to keep my eyes open; I was so tired.

That evening, my own GP rang me to say that he had been contacted by the consultant and that my blood showed that I was very anaemic. He was arranging a blood test for me at the hospital the next day. Mark dropped me off at the hospital. It was a Friday and I told him to go on to work and that I would be all right.

I waited in a wheel chair all day, as this was more comfortable than the ordinary chairs, and felt so weak and worn out that I couldn't even sit in it. I remember shedding a tear on more than one occasion out of sheer hopelessness. I waited and waited. Mark returned from work at the end of the day and I had only just gone in for a blood test and had to wait further to see a doctor. Dr Hailer, a bowel consultant, examined me along with a junior doctor and I was asked many questions. My file was started. He told me that my haemoglobin level was 6 and I distinctly remember him telling me that, if it had been his level, he would be 'flat on the floor'. He was amazed that I had kept going. I had been bleeding from the bowel and he was very concerned when I told him that this had been going on since February 2000. I had seen my GP at the time who had arranged for a barium x-ray to be done. They told me I was fine and had haemorrhoids which were the cause of the bleeding.

Dr Hailer confirmed my problem had been there for a long time from the size of the lump under my chest. He was going to arrange for a blood transfusion straight away and a CT scan in the next few days. I was to stay in hospital for the transfusion.

So much had happened so quickly and I was concerned about school.

'If I feel better after the blood transfusion, can I go to work on Monday?' I asked.

'You won't be going back to work until you see the back of this,' he told me. It was then I started to realise the seriousness of my situation.

That stay in hospital lasted for a week. An ultrasound scan on Monday showed up the tumour in the liver.

'What is the worst thing you fear?' asked the doctor who had to give me the news.

By now, I had already gathered what she was going to tell me; the tumour was 14 by 7 centimetres; this was huge!

'Centimetres or millimetres?' I asked the doctor to confirm. She had to check the notes to inform me it was the former.

I was on my own and had to break the news to Mark when I saw him. Poor Mark had to tell my two sons, Jevan and Aidan, along with the rest of the family who all reacted differently. He told me everything when we met next time. How were Jevan and Aidan? Aidan was away at University in Birmingham. It takes a while for news like this to sink in. It was a complete blow, devastating and difficult to describe the emotions. One day your life continues as normal, the next you are lying in a hospital bed with this outlook. Our life was so lovely; we had everything we needed and were so happy and all that had been turned upside down in an instant.

Mark and I asked so many questions and the doctors were as

helpful as they could be. More tests had to be done. I had to have a CT scan which would be done sooner if I stayed in hospital, so I chose to stay. These scans are so in demand that there is quite a waiting list. I was lucky to slot in for one on Wednesday and awaited the results with trepidation. I asked for these to be checked morning, noon and night but there was no write up on the computer till the next day. The doctor for the Medical Short Stay Unit, where I happened to be, was a wonderful doctor, though I did have a little trouble with his pronunciation. With something like this, you wanted to understand the situation clearly and I asked him to repeat or explain everything as often as I needed.

It was even worse than we thought. Mark was with me, thank goodness, and the doctor left his visit to me until the end of his round of patients. He must have wanted to take all the time needed to deliver this awful news. The tumour in my liver was a secondary and my primary was in the ascending colon. I had terminal cancer.

He looked sadly at us as he talked to us. Mark almost slid off his chair and I remember holding him steady. 'How long has she got?' he asked Dr Harriman.

'Three months, maybe five,' was his answer.

'Is there anything that can be done?' Mark asked.

'Only palliative,' replied Dr Harriman. 'There is no hope.'

Mark totally broke down and I had tears. I thanked the doctor for telling us all this and he left when it was comfortable to do so. Mark and I spent some very precious moments and he held me so tight.

'I don't want to lose you; I don't want to lose you; I can't live without you,' he repeated in floods of tears.

What could I do? What could I say? I told him not to worry. Everything would work out. We spoke about our strength of love for each other and I told Mark how he had given me everything that I wanted. He had to be strong; he was chosen to be Jevan and Aidan's only parent now and I was entrusting him with my most precious gifts in asking him to look after them. He had such a responsibility and something very much to live for.

That night, Mark stayed as long as he could but he did have to get back to tell Jevan and to be with him. He would have to tell Aidan the news over the phone and, of course, Mum and the rest of the family. I didn't envy his task and I'm sure the reality of the situation sank in more and more as he spoke to each one.

I was lucky to have been given a side ward where I was able to be private. I had the urge to write down my thoughts; I didn't want to waste any time. I wrote three letters to Mark, Jevan and Aidan with tears trickling down every now and again. It was so unreal but so real. Then I wrote a poem 'Written on the night I was told there was no hope'. It may all be ending for me but it must go on for everyone else. I wanted others to be happy, not to mourn. I thought about how lucky I actually was, as there was nothing really left undone that I had to do. I had experienced happiness in a wonderful loving marriage which was strong, my two sons were 21 and 19, honest and clever young men, and I was leaving a teaching job that I loved which was sad but meant that I was successful and enjoying what I was doing. I was truly blessed and lucky. So indeed, my poem wasn't miserable but telling people to go on and that my time may have come but we all have to go sometime!

Don't mourn, my darling

(Written on the night I was told there was no hope)
30th November, 2006

Don't mourn, though my body be turned to ashes.
Don't forget my spirit lives on,
And every heart here that interacted with it
Strengthened me.

Don't forget, we all die one day.
And I have died so happy
With a wonderful Mum and Dad, and all my family
So close to me.

How could I wish for more in my life
Than my loving husband and my talented sons?
Don't grieve
I am the luckiest person here.

Don't be negative. I am now wise.
I can tell you that in all my life
I died at my happiest.
Because happiness is created through love.

Be positive then and look forward.
Within your life, see this as a stage
And move on to the next.
And fulfil your dreams.
And above all, be happy,
Love.

Barbara Moss

I put away my A4 pad at last and never looked at it again for over a year. Strangely enough, when I did look at it, I remembered writing the three letters but was surprised to find the poem that I had completely forgotten about!

My family was wonderfully supportive. Mark spent all the time he could with me but I tried to encourage him to try to do normal things like cooking and washing the car. Aidan came back from university and visited me with Jevan. Mum came down from Otley in West Yorkshire and my mother-in-law came over as well. John and Eirian, my brother and sister-in-law came from Ledbury and also Margaret, my sister, who lived locally. My brother, Peter, also from Otley, was not able to come away and sent his wishes. I was so conscious of upsetting all these people and taking up their time but I was happy to see them all and to know that they cared.

It's a strange thing, I suppose. What do people talk about in these circumstances? I can remember a funny incident one Sunday morning when it's quiet in the hospital. The doctors don't do routine rounds and so on. A large car had tried to 'escape' paying the parking charges and, while the car park was relatively empty, had tried to drive across the raised paving to get out of the car park rather than go through the barrier and pay. The driver got his front wheels over the ridge but then became stuck with his rear wheels wedged behind. The middle of the car was sitting on the raised area with the front and rear wheels on either side of it and the driver couldn't move it! It was there for a while until the culprit returned with two hefty men in black suits who lifted up the rear and pushed him out. There was a nasty large puddle left behind which looked suspiciously like oil. I was able to tell all my visitors about this and we laughed, which was what I wanted to do.

I also wanted to do normal things. I asked for my laptop and wrote lesson plans for school as I felt so guilty leaving them so abruptly. I was so fortunate in having planned major pieces of work, which I had word processed and copied in readiness. I only had to leave instructions for these to be handed to many of my classes and the children could carry on with the work. I spent time preparing worksheets for my GCSE class and Jevan e-mailed all this to school.

Friday morning, a week after receiving the dreadful news, I had a visit from Dr Hailer who told me that there was an MDT meeting at lunchtime. This is a Mixed Disciplinary Team Meeting which happens at lunchtime as this is the only time in common the doctors have the opportunity to meet. There would be consultants from different fields as well as a palliative nurse and other support staff. Dr Hailer informed me that my condition was to be discussed that day and he would make a point of seeing me before his afternoon appointments, which started at two o'clock. Mark and I waited as the time ticked by so slowly from one thirty. It seemed like forever to hear the outcome of this meeting. It was almost two when Dr Hailer arrived, out of breath. He sat on the edge of the bed and looked straight at me. The liver surgeon from The Queen Elizabeth Hospital in Birmingham happened to be at that meeting. He is only able to attend about once a month but, to my luck, he was there today. He said that if the tumour could shrink, he was prepared to operate and remove it. My condition hadn't changed but what a difference this made. There was something to aim for! There was hope!

2 *My Diagnosis*

When I returned home, which was lovely, the familiar things around me all seemed different somehow. I started to look closely at objects that had always been there and taken for granted; the furniture, the carpet and curtains, the pictures on the wall. I started to see things I hadn't seen before. I also felt prominent in myself and conscious of my body; instead of just being there, I was the centre of attention. This was, of course, because everyone was caring for me but I must say it felt odd. Both the schools where I worked had sent me enormous bouquets of flowers and numerous cards. I had been sent so many wishes and very kind words were said about me and my work. I felt truly loved and all this helped me so much. I cannot describe in words the amount of strength I received through the prayers that were being said for me. I felt a wall around me that made me secure and unafraid: I couldn't ask for more of life and felt completely at peace.

I had been given an appointment to see Dr Farrago, who was to be my consultant, that Tuesday afternoon. Mark and I waited a long time; he was running very late but he always spent as long as he needed with each patient, never rushing anybody. This was reassuring for us. Dr Farrago made no promises but helped us to understand exactly what the plan was. He booked me in to have a PICC line inserted in my arm through which the chemotherapy drugs would be administered. This saves the necessity of a large needle, called a canula, being inserted each time one has treatment. My appointment was made for my first chemotherapy after that but, first, I was to have a colonoscopy where a camera is inserted up the bowel and a biopsy of the tumour is taken to determine the nature of the cancer.

The colonoscopy was done by Dr Hailer at Kidderminster Hospital. He told me that if he found any polyps, he would slice them off if I agreed to this. This is how cancer starts in the bowel. I was quite nervous, wondering whether something up the lower end was indeed any easier than something down the top! I was told that I would be given oxygen and some sort of local pain relief. In situations like these, you just have to lie there and let be done what has to be done. You don't watch and your dignity is maintained as much as possible. There was a small monitor that showed you the inside of the bowel as the camera travelled through. There were obviously twists and turns inside and each of these required an extra shove of the camera. I know that I groaned and Dr Hailer asked the nurse whether any more anaesthetic could be administered. I was allowed a little bit more. I'm not sure whether I actually felt any less discomfort but just knowing that I was given more was a big help! I was completely alert and aware of what was happening. This process continued for a while when suddenly Dr Hailer called out loudly, 'There it is!' I could see it clearly on the screen: small speckled fatty looking things with points, clinging to the inside skin of the bowel in a ring. The doctor was obviously quite excited at this point and I was wide awake now. He projected a little instrument inside me which pinched a piece of tissue from several of these horrible looking fatty things and a drop of blood trickled out each time on the screen. This bit was not painful and I found it quite interesting. Removing the camera was quick and not too bad. After this, I had to rest and eat a sandwich before being allowed to go home. Mark waited by my side, sensitive to everything I was going through. I always thought that witnessing this was far worse than having to experience it oneself.

The results showed that I had bowel cancer as expected and chemotherapy could now proceed.

3 *Preparing for Christmas*

I was to have a PICC line inserted before Christmas and my first chemo on January the second. The PICC line was a very fine tube that had to travel through a vein from the inside elbow, across the shoulder and stop at an accurate point to deliver the drugs where they would mix with your blood and travel around the body. My right arm had the better vein to use and I had to wedge my head to the right, which helped prevent the tube from travelling upwards towards the head when it passed across the shoulder. A quick x-ray showed that it was in the right position. Thank goodness! Otherwise the whole thing had to be done again.

Preparation for Christmas went on as normally as possible with the shopping and so on done. Mark was always given a fresh turkey by his company and he brought this home as usual. Aidan was back from University and Mum was still with us. A couple of days before the big day, my right arm became hot and ached. The PICC line had turned red and hot up to my shoulder and was swollen. We were quite worried and phoned the helpline we had been given at Cheltenham Hospital. I had been told that I must ring them rather than go to the GP as the latter would be inclined to remove the line as a first resort. The hospital wanted me in straight away and so Mark and I packed the bag and he drove me there, about thirty miles away. We waited several hours to be seen and then I was told that I would have to stay in to have a treatment of strong antibiotics intravenously. I was, of course, down about having to stay in hospital again. Poor Mark had to return home on his own and get on with everything that I had planned, but without me. On top of everything else, this must have been so difficult.

Mark and Mum visited me every day along with Jevan and Aidan on several occasions. This is where Bobby 'was born'. Mark brought me this beautiful blue wheat bear that you could warm up in the microwave; it took two minutes and the heat relieved the pain in my arm. I called him Bobbles because of his bobble tail, but Bobby for short! To this day, Bobby has stayed with me every day and has accompanied us on all our numerous memorable trips in the caravan. He has developed an inquisitive personality, asking many questions which highlight the ambiguity of our language. He's a teddy that makes you smile and he's been a wonderful little friend. Bobby now looks much loved with his lilac ribbon very frayed around his neck.

A few days passed but the hope of coming out of hospital before Christmas dwindled as I had a temperature; they did, however, let me go home for the afternoon on Christmas Day. Mark came all that way to collect me. When I got home, everything was laid out ready and beautiful. There were carols playing and the table looked wonderful with crackers and serviettes. A lovely smell of Christmas dinner was coming from the kitchen. I was going to try a new recipe, just cooking the turkey breast with onions, butter and garlic. Jevan and Aidan did all this instead of me; they cooked the parsnips with parmesan and the little sausages with bacon. They did everything perfectly. It was lovely. I enjoyed the meal tremendously and then sat on the settee with my feet up, a sight everyone has got so used to seeing now! I felt so cold and Mark brought me an orange blanket. We opened our presents and thanked each other.

Everyone had waited for me. Time passed very quickly and it was soon time to return to the hospital, a bit like Cinderella! I had to be back for a certain time to have my antibiotics. I was really shivering so I took the blanket in the car, finding it difficult to even sit on the seat. My temperature had shot up and I felt dreadfully ill.

My brother John and his wife, Eirian, had arranged a get-together a couple of days after Christmas. I was really looking forward to this and the hope was that I would be out of hospital by then. I knew that the whole thing was quite special for me though this may seem to be a conceited view. Before my illness, the family was not able to find a date suitable for all but everyone had made a special effort now. I was feeling so much better. Alas, my temperature would not return to normal and, though it was only slightly up, I was not allowed out. I was really, really disappointed but told Mark to go to the get-together with Jevan, Aidan and Mum. They all came to visit me first and Mum brought me some beautiful lizzyanthemums which Mark put in a vase. I was convinced that my temperature was only due to the fact that I had not been having my paracetamol which I had been taking at home. I asked to see Dr Farrago and he did come over. He joked at me saying, 'What are you doing here?'

'I want to go home,' I replied and I was delighted when he told me that I could. Poor Mark drove back all the way from John's to pick me up and take me home but he was pleased to have me back. I thoroughly enjoyed the biryani and samba that Eirian had sent for me and ate it straight away.

The next day, Margaret, my sister, had prepared a special buffet lunch for the whole family and again, everyone had waited for me to be there to exchange and open presents. I had a wonderful time and appreciated this so much. Peter, my younger brother, and his family were able to stay for this before returning home to Otley. It was a very special occasion and I enjoyed it tremendously.

Returning home after all this made me feel much loved and I also felt that my illness had brought the family together. The effect of this unity gave me so much strength and I didn't feel afraid at all.

4 *The First Chemo*

I was visited by Marilyn, the Macmillan nurse after this and she was the most fabulous woman, cheerful and so down to earth. She booked me in to visit St Richard's Hospice for the terminally ill and advised on many things. She was surprised that Mark and I had already done so much. With the help of the bursar at school, I had made arrangements to retire early on the grounds of ill health and swift action here saved me a great deal of money. Terms for pensions were changing in the New Year. Mark and I had also made an appointment with solicitors to renew our will in the light of current circumstances. It was important to be careful and without being ruthless, it was important to recognise and ensure what I would want for Jevan and Aidan, my two sons. It is important to say here that for Mark and me it was our second marriage and Jevan and Aidan are my two sons.

Mark and I had also applied for whatever we were entitled to regarding Disability Living Allowances and obtained a Blue Badge to make outings easier. Marilyn was going to do all this for us but it had been done!

Marilyn made several more visits at regular intervals and she always made us feel good. If I needed any medication, she rang the doctor's immediately and arranged it straight away. There was one occasion when Mark and I felt on edge with each other and we asked Marilyn to discuss it with us. I had felt quite strong up to now but the bickering at this time was getting me down and making me cry. It was strange because Mark felt that I wasn't coping and I felt that it was him. Talking about it openly was what we needed because Marilyn didn't tell us anything new but she helped us by listening and after this we had no more problems like this. Mark has been a terrific strength, coping with me and his work throughout. I never took any of this for granted; I was indeed blessed.

I had been nervous that my first chemotherapy would be delayed but I was lucky that all the swelling in my arm had gone down. Mum was still with us and came with me for the treatment and Mark was always by my side. Bobby was always there and Mum kept warming him up for me. I was seen by Dr Farrago first and after that, had to wait a long time for the drugs to arrive. They could not be dispensed until the doctor had given the go-ahead because of their cost. I also had to have a blood test to show that I was fit enough to have these toxic drugs. My appointment was for nine thirty and I was not finished until five o'clock. It was a long day and I marvelled at the chemo nurses in The Rowan Suite of Worcester Royal. They were all so cheerful and there was a volunteer, Annie, who came round, chatted to you and brought you coffee. Everyone was so friendly. I remember thinking that they must be specially chosen.

Hannah was my nurse and she explained what each drug was and what she was going to do. I had to have three different drugs with saline between each one, all administered intravenously. Before any of this, I was given anti-sickness drugs in the same way; one of these was a steroid to make the others work better. My chemotherapy was to be oxalyplatin 5FU every fortnight. As it passed through, I felt sick and my eyes and lips twitched. It tasted of chemicals, sickly sweet. You smelt it and you smelt of it. The 5FU was taken over forty-eight hours so I was able to have this hanging on a bag with a little electronic gadget which would bleep if there was any blockage. When I left the hospital I noticed the effects of the oxalyplatin. It made ordinary cold feel like sub-zero. A glass of water felt ice cold to the extent it was uncomfortable to hold. Outside, the cold breeze of the darkening day froze against my face and I was actually scarred through frost bite for quite a while by this. I was very careful the next time to cover my face and Mark picked me up outside the hospital door from then on.

I felt really tired for the rest of the evening and, indeed, for the next few days. I had a regular rest each day in the afternoon and frequent rests in-between. I was really spoilt with everyone else doing the cooking and bringing me whatever I needed and didn't need! Mum helped so much. When I could, I was walking around with all these thin tubes everywhere and it was interesting trying to get dressed or have a shower. Mark had to hold the bottle outside the cubicle while I did what I could. Showering was so important as the cancer made me sweat so much at night. The sheets were soaked and I had to lay towels under me and change them in the night. Things like this just happened and you put up with it. Complaining about it never entered my head; it was part of the illness and everything possible was being done to help me.

I had a District Nurse visit me between each treatment and she removed the 5FU bottle and did a blood test. I got very used to all the needles and this wasn't a problem. The bloods were tested for haemoglobin which was low for me because I was losing so much blood. The white blood cells were important because this showed your resistance to infection. These were fast dividing cells, so they were killed back by the chemo drugs. If these were too low you became neutropenic and this was a dangerous situation because one would be unable to fight even a minor infection such as a cold. I also had a CEA test which showed tumour activity by measuring protein levels in the blood. My reading was 38 and I understood that below 5 was normal. I got to know all the District Nurses really well. They were all lovely, happy, kind and friendly and work all hours of the day even though many have young families of their own. I marvelled at how special these people were; they didn't just do a difficult job, they had to be so patient and kind, always.

I returned home with all the anti-sickness tablets and instructions. Mum had cooked a lovely fish molee, something to help me gain an appetite. I did my best to eat a little but as the evening grew, I felt more and more sick and went upstairs. I was violently ill and felt helpless, unable to control anything and having to sit on the floor next to the toilet. I was told to expect to feel ill but if this continued I was to phone the helpline at Cheltenham. We felt it best to phone the hospital and again, I had to go in and there was Mark taking me. I was monitored and stabilised for a few days and things settled after that. I felt such a nuisance to everyone as I was causing so much disruption; they were flooding me with their love and I was giving them nothing back in return.

Mum stayed all this time and continued to do whatever she could to help; lots of cooking and keeping me company, bringing me drinks and warming up Bobby. She always said her prayers each morning as did both the schools where I worked and friends and relatives around the globe. I certainly felt the strength that these prayers gave me; something was helping me to face my illness and to fight it.

About ten days after the chemo, I had a very low period in which I felt particularly tired. I didn't even feel like getting out of bed so having Mum there actually gave me an incentive to get up, although I just lay on the couch most of the day. This lasted for about three days and is called the 'nadir'. I understand that your white blood cells are particularly low at this time, meaning that your resistance to fighting infection is low. One is just picking up when it's time to be knocked down again by the next chemo!

It was soon time for the second chemo; I had to have them every two weeks; the same process. I waited to see Dr Farrago who checked side effects and how I had reacted to the chemo. He was a wonderful man and gave his time readily. He was happy for me to have my chemo as the bloods had been fine. The drugs can knock your neutrophils down to such an extent that you have no immunity and then chemotherapy has to be delayed. I did have problems with my haemoglobin on several occasions; I had lost so much blood that I became anaemic nearly every fortnight and had to have a transfusion before my chemo each time. After quite a few of these, Dr Farrago arranged for me to see a specialist to apply some radiotherapy to the colon. I do remember this experience vividly as Mark had to take me to Cheltenham every day for a week. It was even more unfortunate as it was the week of the Gold Cup and the traffic was horrendous; still Mark never complained or even minded. On arriving back home, he went on to work and filled his day. The radiotherapy did have the desired effect; my bleeding stopped. However, I was left with acute pain in my lower abdomen where the treatment may have caught an area that it shouldn't have. It is quite interesting how the exact spot is measured and dots placed on your body so that the location is targeted accurately each time. I was limping around for several weeks before this eased but I was so pleased that I did not have to have any more transfusions after this.

I had now got to know many of the nurses and also some of the patients I had seen from the previous time at Worcester. I introduced myself to them and they all did the same and I remember saying it was like 'Groundhog Day'. It made the situation more relaxed and we got to know each other better in future weeks. There was one poor lady who had advanced bowel cancer and she just didn't want to know anything about her treatment or condition. She just did as instructed and on talking to her, I learned that her husband had been diagnosed with leukaemia the previous year. There were so many people in a far worse situation than mine.

5 St. Richard's Hospice, Worcester

Mum returned to Otley after a long stay and I arranged to go to St Richard's Hospice for terminally ill patients. Mark and I were invited to visit the hospice together before I decided to join the day centre. St Richard's moved to a lovely new building a few years ago, just around the corner from our house. It is set in beautiful grounds next to the Country Park and Nunnery Wood. I was very impressed with the atmosphere and all the facilities available to me there. I was greeted by Collette, one of the nurses, and she showed me around the day centre, mainly a large day room overlooking the garden and a large dining room. There were also several small side rooms, where we talked about what I could gain from the hospice. There was a room with a large bath and a chapel which was called the 'Quiet Room'; this had a beautiful stained glass window, a few chairs and a small table altar to one side. What really impressed me was the relaxed, content atmosphere within; everyone seemed happy though here was a group of patients, all of whom were terminally ill. Some were doing craftwork or painting, a couple were working on a jigsaw, some were sitting in a group and talking, others were lying quietly with their eyes closed, perhaps asleep. On this day, many of the patients were quite elderly but I was told that on Wednesdays the group was quite mixed.

I arranged to go every other week on a Wednesday but once I

had been there, I went every week! There was a hairdresser, Tracy, who was a really good stylist. She worked in the morning on a Wednesday, giving up her time freely to help others like me. Tracy had a sister who had died of cancer in Spain. There were so many other volunteers. Nina treated me to some reflexology. She was quite amazing and when she pressed the nerves on my foot, I could feel the corresponding part of the body that it applied to. She asked me where I felt the pinging and it was correct. I felt very tired after the reflexology and, on my way home, had palpitations in my colon. This showed how powerful the treatment was but I felt that, because of the chemotherapy, I had better leave this as it was too strong for me. The next time I tried Reiki. I had always thought that this would be useless as you weren't even touched. However, I felt so relaxed and heavenly after this and have been lucky enough to be offered this treatment several times. Lunch was a grand occasion and the volunteers served us a choice between a meat and vegetarian meal. The tables were beautifully laid with tablecloths and a centrepiece of flowers, always fresh. In the afternoon, I chose to go to 'Quiet Time'. This was just a quiet session usually held in the chapel; sometimes there would be prayer or communion, other times we talked, read poetry or listened to music. I always enjoyed these times; being there with people who truly understood meant so much to me and helped me.

I have grown to look forward to these days at St Richard's; I have learned so much from the people there, both patients and volunteers and I have realised just how lucky I am to be still around. So many of the friends I have made have passed away, many of them younger than me. It makes no difference who you are or how rich you may be when life is taken. Talking to all these people and remembering them has helped me; we often talked about death and how the family would accept it. It sounds morose but it helps one to be able to talk to people who understand and are going through the same. Other friends often find it too upsetting to talk in the way we could; they find it hard to see how we could be so open. I had got to know Delia so well and she told me about the cardboard coffin with poppies around the side that she had ordered for herself over the internet. It is very hard when you actually see the coffin in the church and think back to the conversation that we had. It was impossible to really imagine her active body so lifeless as she lay there.

6 *Recap on Living Life*

I had tolerated a couple of chemos and had learned what to expect. I told Mark to leave me after I had seen Dr Farrago but he always came to collect me when I was done. I phoned him just before I was ready and he would be there within minutes. Mark cared for me, bringing my footstool and blanket and a glass of water. The drugs weakened and tired me dreadfully but I knew it would pass in time again. We felt confident after a while to take a trip out in our caravan. We had a free holiday for ten days during the Easter break on a campsite at Bath Marina. This had been given to us because of help I had given the organisation the previous year. This was the only booking I had not cancelled as it was not going to cost us anything. We eagerly got the caravan ready for the trip, ticking our prepared lists and adding several items and medications I may need. I found the nearest hospital in case of emergency and also made arrangements to have my PICC line flushed there. This had to be done in between chemos to ensure it did not get blocked. It just meant that some saline was passed through with a syringe to keep it flowing. We arranged to have a pitch next to the toilet block to make things easier for me. We had been to this site before and it is very pretty; we knew the layout of the pitches and so we felt confident to go there.

Mark and I felt very excited when we arrived in Bath. I don't

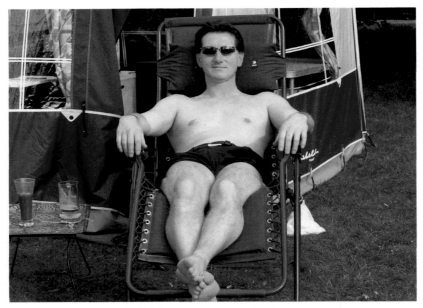

Bath Marina campsite in April 2007

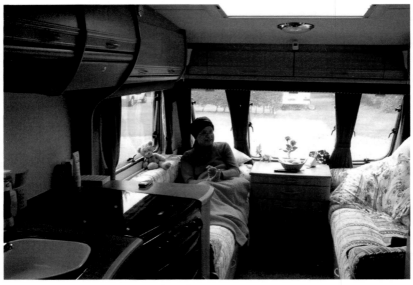

'Summer's Wood' campsite in May 2007

think we really expected to be going out in our caravan ever again. This was such a treat and Mark did not mind doing all the setting up which included erecting the awning on his own. I remember doing a couple of little things but Mark insisted on me resting after the journey.

It was wonderful, feeling the freedom of sitting in the van when all was done and feeling proud. In fact, we even went into the city for a little while that afternoon just to feel we had done something. We developed a pattern of going out in the morning and returning for a rest in the afternoon. Mark would get out the pillows and blanket and I often slept for a couple of hours during which time Mark played his guitar outside and sang. This has remained the pattern we have followed on numerous trips since then.

I felt that I was getting better and, after my fourth chemo, I was due a CT scan. This is a CAT scan which looks like a giant polo mint through which you pass while lying down. It takes numerous photos of your internal organs in 3D layers so that any section can be looked at as a plate. In this way, the tumours can be seen and measured so that the effect of the chemotherapy can be seen. For scans involving the bowel, however, you have to drink 600ml of this awful orange aniseedy stuff at ten o'clock the night before and then a litre of gungy gluey white stuff one hour before the scan. The quantity is quite scary but amazingly enough, you get through it if you don't think about it too much. Before the scan, a canula is placed in your vein for a contrast solution to be passed through during the scan itself. This is quite peculiar as it feels very warm when this happens and you think you're wetting yourself. Anyway, this was all done and I looked forward to the results.

I remember that day vividly. Dr Farrago wasn't there so I saw Dr Steel, a member of Dr. Farrago's team. Mark was with me, of course. He told us it was bad news and I really could not believe I was hearing those words. The tumour in the liver had, in fact, grown and the chemo wasn't working. He said that my CEA level had increased to 38 from a starting point of about 16. This was an indicator of what was happening as it showed tumour activity by measuring the protein in the blood. The tumour was now fifteen by ten centimetres, the size of a grapefruit. The outlook was not good; if my prognosis was three to five months before, what was it now? Dr Steel explained with diagrams how tumours can spread; you could have a large mass or several small lumps. My chemo was to be changed and I was put on irinotecan, a different drug, along with the 5FU as before. There was a fifty-fifty chance of this drug working, only the same as before. I had to give it a try but, with this drug, I was going to lose my hair and I wasn't looking forward to the prospect of this.

I had the chemo, twitching even more and hating its foul taste. It formed a wet layer on the inside of my nose and if I sniffed, the liquid would trickle down my throat. The only consolation was that this chemo would be every three weeks. I suffered more side effects with this one but didn't get the freezing sensations. The day came and went. I was determined to get to that operating table!

This almost happened sooner than expected! Dr Farrago had warned me that if my stomach swelled up, I should contact accident and emergency; this could happen if the growing tumour in the colon caused a blockage and this is what seemed to be happening to me. We rang A&E and had to go straight in. I was placed in a side room immediately and I can say that I was looked after really well. I had quite a temperature but kept my little cap on for fear of messing up the sheets with my falling hair. The lovely nurse encouraged me to remove the cap, telling me not to worry about the bits of hair; that was not a problem.

I had the usual checks and one for diabetes which, I was told, was now routinely done at A&E. I was soon seen by a doctor but I was in terrible pain and requested a laxative; this was not given to me, in fact, till the end of the day as I was informed that an emergency operation to remove the tumour in the bowel was likely. I didn't want this to happen as I wanted both tumours removed together, as planned; I knew that this would give me the best chance of survival. My stomach continued to swell and I was getting more and more uncomfortable. Eventually I was given a bed in one of the wards, the MSSU or Medical Short Stay Unit. I was given some soup and hoped that the bowel would free itself after being given some ghastly, sickly sweet medicine that tasted like thick glycerine.

I shared the bay with three other women but I really wasn't in a mood to make polite conversation. However, the next morning I had the wonderful feeling of severe stomach ache and visited the bathroom attached to our bay. It made the whole ward laugh when they heard me singing 'Alleluia' at the top of my voice! I would now be able to return home after the doctor's check and now, no emergency op.

7 *June 2007, Mixed Blessings*

Hannah gave me a voucher from the hospital for a free wig. I looked up the shop website in Bromsgrove and made an appointment before my hair started to fall too much. I chose a style closest to the previous length and colour of my hair, together with all the shampoo and conditioner I would need to look after the wig. It was an interesting experience and Mark was very helpful in telling me how each one looked.

After the second of the new treatments, my hair started to fall in chunks. When I ran the comb through it, a large chunk of hair came with it. I decided to have it cut short to lessen the shock when I would have none left; later on, I actually had it shaved off completely. The annoyance of picking up hairs from the bedclothes was greater than the horrible aspect of having no hair. I went to the barber's with Mark and asked them to shave my head. I don't suppose they were presented with a woman's head too often but the dear barber who did this didn't mind. He told me that the last time he had done this was for his wife who died of cancer some years ago; it must have brought back some memories for the dear man. After this, I was, in fact, much more able to cope with my head. I had bought a very pretty brown broderie anglaise bonnet from the wig shop and this was comfortable and fashionable to wear instead of the wig when it was hot. Everyone admired it.

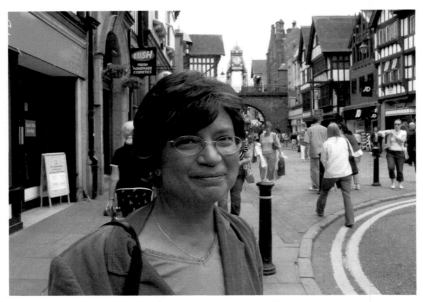

Me and my Wig. June 2007 Chester

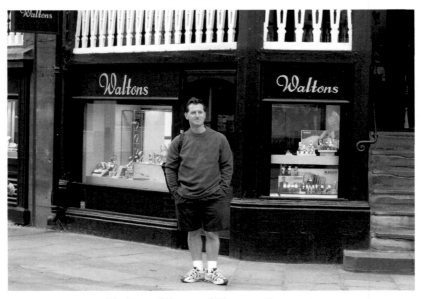

The beautiful town of Chester in June 2007

Three weeks between chemos gave Mark and me more time to get away and we planned as many trips out in our caravan as we could. We always checked for the nearest hospital, taking a 'hospital bag' in case of emergency and we went to places from which we could get back to Cheltenham quickly if the need arose. We went to some of our favourite haunts, to Oxford and Cirencester.

In the summer we were a little more adventurous and went to Nottingham, a place we hadn't stayed at before. We were allowed a good pitch that had been out of commission because of the huge amount of recent rain; it had therefore not been allocated to anyone. Although this campsite wasn't up to the standard we usually looked for, the people we met were fantastic. They would sing along to Mark's playing and shout out requests. They asked us over for a drink on our last night and said that they wanted to see me again the next year. They told us which pitch was best for the sun and the warden got his little tractor to help pull our caravan out of our pitch because it had a tight turning space.

There was a young family on the site who I will never forget; they were so amazing. The parents were quite young and had four children, twin lads of about nine, a younger girl and a little girl who had MS and confined to a wheelchair. She had no use of her legs and arms. What was truly amazing was that they were camping in a tent. The little girl had to be carried in and out of the tent and placed in her wheelchair. They managed marvellously and were always happy. It makes you wonder when people complain about minor ailments how a family like this just got on and coped and had fun.

I was experiencing several headaches at this time and Dr Farrago, always cautious, arranged for me to have a head scan. This was clear but because of continued pains in my shoulder and back, he arranged a bone scan after this. I was keen to get the results and during my appointment before the chemo, asked him for these. He phoned for them to be faxed through and received them at the very end of my meeting with him. 'It says, "Extensive metastases of the bone",' he told me directly. All my hopes and lifted spirits felt as though a lead weight had suddenly been dropped on them.

'Does it say where?' I asked but it didn't and I could see his concern. He discussed radiation treatment, asking me where I had got pains and so on. I was, of course, completely knocked back and was very quiet that day for my chemotherapy. The nurses knew me well and respected my desire to remain quiet with the occasional tear I could not prevent. I had to tell Mark, as yet, and he was at work. During his lunchtime, I phoned him to give him this bad news; we understood what this meant and my hopes for a cure were fast fading.

Dr Farrago spent his entire lunchtime meeting the radiologist who did the scan report in order to examine the scan and see what was going on. He returned to see me in the afternoon while my chemo was still going on; I was going to be finished in about half an hour so he thought it best to wait till then so he could give me some privacy but he told me that he had some news on the report. Imagine my delight when he explained that an error had been made. The reports are recorded on a Dictaphone and on pressing the button to record, the word 'No' had not recorded. The report should have said, 'NO extensive metastases of the bone'. I had no cancer in the bone. Dr Farrago had examined the scans in depth with the radiologist and they could find no evidence of any bone cancer. Of course, I had an apology but I was ecstatic and couldn't wait to phone Mark which I did the moment I stepped out of the hospital doors. The only thing I asked was for Dr Farrago to get a written explanation of this mistake in order to prevent future errors such as this.

Time was passing and I was due a CT scan after four of the new treatments. I started to feel a huge improvement in the liver; the lump felt much smaller. I had been unable to sleep on my stomach before as it hurt my chest and the lump weighed heavy when I turned in bed; now that was easing and I felt it lighter as I turned over. I was cautious about what to expect, however, after my previous experience. I spoke to Dr Farrago about all this and he asked to examine me. He agreed; the lump had measured four fingers from top to bottom, now it measured only three. This was marvellous and gave us all renewed hope that I would be able to have an operation. My scan was planned after the fourth chemo and then an appointment made with Mr Broomhall, who would be my surgeon at the Queen Elizabeth Hospital in Birmingham.

I had my scan, not worrying as much about the horrible drink I had to take this time because of the anticipation of what the results could mean. However, the physical effects of this drink, loosening the bowel even more than the chemo had already done could not be ignored! I went to see Dr Farrago for the results the next week and he looked happy. He congratulated me and Mark was so delighted. The lump had shrunk by 25 percent in both directions. This was surely a miracle! My appointment was made to see Mr Broomhall and within a few days Mark took me up to Birmingham to meet him. I remember my first impressions of him and thinking that this was the genius who would be totally entrusted with my life: he was a butcher of a man, towering, broad shouldered and spoke with a gruff but kind voice. He had a big smile on his face and I immediately liked him.

Simon Broomhall looked directly at me when he spoke. He tried to get up the actual scan for me to see; Mark and I had actually seen this before as we had asked Dr Farrago to see it and he set it up for us on his monitor. He told me that I had had wonderful results but unfortunately, there was still further to go. Whilst the tumour had shrunk significantly, it was in the left lobe of the liver and it was too close to the portal vein. This vein would need to be left intact during the operation when the left lobe was removed. There were three veins to the left lobe and the other two could be removed with no problem; the tumour not only had to shrink more but it had to shrink away from the portal vein. We saw all the scans and could see how the tumour became elongated when it touched this important vein; if the tumour was to be removed, there would have to be clearance with healthy cells which could be cut away. We talked about the best treatments and he told us that he would recommend Avastin, a new type of treatment, along with conventional chemotherapy. Mark and I left feeling terribly, terribly disappointed; this was such a journey. However, I had got this far and there was no giving up or turning back now.

8 *Am I Worth it?*

Mark and I had read about Erbitux and Avastin. By sheer chance, one of Mum's friends had seen an article in Saga Magazine about a man suffering advanced bowel cancer in America and had been treated with Erbitux; he had reacted amazingly well to it. Mum sent me this article and after that we researched quite a lot about these treatments. These drugs were grouped as monoclonal antibodies and were already being used widely in America and Europe. They work by targeting the cancer cells and capping them, starving them of oxygen or food. Because they are cloned from one cell, they work in the same way with all cancer cells of that type. If the treatment works for you at all, it will work well. These treatments are quite different from chemotherapy, which targets all cells that divide, hence all the side effects of killing your white blood cells and losing your hair. We were very interested in discussing this with Dr Farrago but there was one drawback; these drugs were not freely available on the NHS; they were private and had to be paid for at great expense. Furthermore, by opting to have what might be your life saver, you were immediately excluded from the treatment you were currently having on the NHS. Mum immediately said that if we opted for any of these treatments, she would pay for half of all the costs and she kept to her word throughout, backing us and encouraging us in our decisions.

My appointment with Dr Farrago left us feeling very positive. I chose to have Avastin and he said that he recommended it alongside irinotecan with 5FU which could be taken as tablets. These were taken for fourteen days following the chemo and then a rest for seven days before the next treatment. I was to have a scan after the third treatment and an appointment with Simon Broomhall after the fourth with a view to the op. I was to be given another chance and these new drugs sounded so good if they worked for you that I was looking forward to the results even though I wasn't looking forward to the treatment. The four treatments along with payment for Dr Farrago's care and cost of the hospital room were going to cost £10,500. My emotions were tossed up and down; I wanted the treatment but was I worth all this money? Surely it was better to leave it for the living!

Mark had no doubt that we were going to do all we could. He told me not to even think about the cost. Dr Farrago applied to the NHS for funding for me but this was refused. What a system we lived in; Scotland and Wales were using these drugs without any problems. Some authorities were granting them more readily than others. Worcestershire was not budging.

We continued to have our breaks as often as we could between each treatment and met so many wonderful people every time. All this helped and there was always something to look forward to, which made such a difference. The only thing that was difficult was to book anything in advance. We always had to see how I was after the chemo which was now having an accumulative effect; some of the symptoms were getting worse and I was getting cramps in the abdomen more often and having to visit the toilet a few times each day. There was also the problem that, if chemo was postponed because of the bloods, I would be a week or two out for any booking; thus we waited patiently each time and made plans very quickly if all appeared well.

9 *New Hope*

I continued to go to St Richard's and always looked forward to this. David, the chaplain of the hospice had shown a group of us some paintings by Michel Petrone. Michel had died of cancer earlier in the year after a long battle for survival and during a period of respite, his girlfriend also died of the disease. He had painted a series of pictures which described his journey and we talked about what he must have felt at each point. They were wonderful and had been published in an important health magazine, The Lancet, to help specialists to understand what cancer sufferers experience. I was so inspired by these paintings that I looked up information about Michel Petrone on the internet when I got home. There was plenty to be found, along with his explanations to each painting. It was so interesting to compare our own interpretations with his descriptions. Michel had started a website of his own and invited other people to send in their paintings with a story attached to each.

I decided that I would like to express my feelings too and when Bridie, specialist in arts and crafts at the hospice, asked me whether I would like to paint, I must have shocked her with my reply. But what would I paint? That morning I had some reiki and the thoughts came flooding. I couldn't wait to start. There was one problem; I couldn't draw! 'But people could only laugh if it was awful,' I thought. I had never been any good at art in school and dropped the subject at the age of twelve. It took several visits to St Richard's before the painting made progress. I talked to people too much about what I was doing and what it meant and didn't put enough time into the task. Deidre said that I should have it next to my bed when I go for the operation. People kept commenting about the 'hand' picture and who had done it. Anyway, I finished it and here it is.

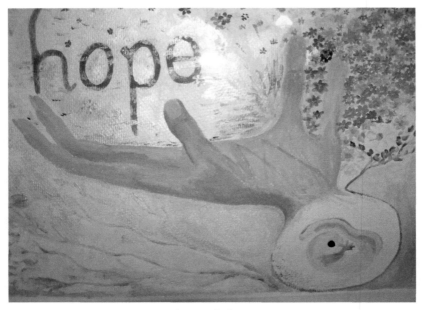

The Hand of Hope

Mark was very proud of it and Aidan was surprised when he saw it. 'I thought it would be rubbish,' he said, 'but it's good.' Mum asked me to write an explanation of it and this is what I wrote:

THE HAND OF HOPE

Here I am as an embryo, surrounded by love, warmth, care, and feeling completely safe. I am given all the nourishment that I need. I have no fears of what may happen; I know that it is all part of a plan and I accept it.

However, an embryo will grow into a strong, independent person and that is my hope. The hand represents me reaching out for this and the long fingers are stretched as far as they can go. The large palm accepts gratefully all the help that is given, not an easy task to keep taking, and it also shows acceptance of my illness. You can see that the back of the hand completely holds down the starkness of the bare branches encrusted in ice. This represents my cancer and what has to be fought.

There is an abundance of joy, peculiar to think, but there is a joy you experience in my condition that would not otherwise happen. It stems from a complete peace of mind. This can be seen by the flowers clustered to the right of the hand and as they flutter in the breeze, they whisper, 'Catch me if you can!'

10 *Hope, Faith and Maybe*

I must say that Bobby was well travelled for a little bear. He sat in the caravan on each of our journeys and started to look as though he had been around for a while. He was getting extremely chatty and became part of the family. My hair started to fall again; it had been growing a little but with the new course of chemo, it started to fall. I promptly had it shaved off this time and felt happier for this.

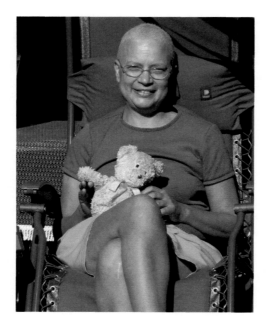

My fourth chemo completed the course prescribed by Dr Farrago who warned me that 'getting to the operation was one thing; getting through it was another'. He wanted me to know that there were many risks such as infection or reaction to the anaesthetic. We now awaited news from Mr Broomhall, my surgeon. Mark and I decided to go to Newent, on the edge of the Forest of Dean, for a short stay. It was a really beautiful place and the campsite was unique. It was the weekend of the famous 'onion fair' which takes place on the second Saturday in September. It was so much fun as the lovely village was decorated and all the shops had onion figures in the windows; the travel agents had onions with faces, lying on sun beds and opticians had onions wearing glasses. Mr Broomhall was to contact me with the results. If I needed more chemo, we would return in time for this.

My mobile was switched on and kept within reach; I dashed outside when it rang to get the best reception. Mr. Broomhall was such a jolly man and told me that my reaction to Avastin had been amazing and that he was happy to operate. He said, 'Don't have any more chemo; enjoy your holiday' and 'I'll see you on the Friday before your operation'. This was pencilled in for October the fourth and to be confirmed in writing. October the fourth was the optimum time for the operation as it would be six weeks after my last chemo. One of the side effects of Avastin is that it prevents blood from clotting. It is not possible, therefore, to operate until these effects have had time to wear off which takes six weeks. We were over the moon and went to the proprietor of the campsite who understood our situation; her husband had suddenly died of cancer two years ago. She was so happy for us and allowed us to extend our stay by three days as we did not now have to return for treatment. Within fifteen minutes, the news had spread over the whole campsite and we had numerous people coming over to us to share our joy.

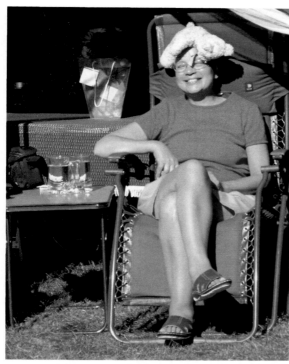

Who needs a wig?

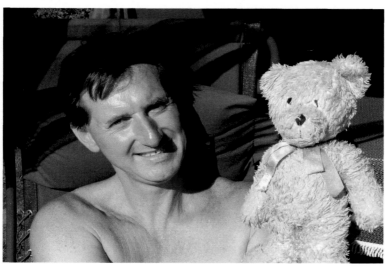

The next week, Mark and I went to see Simon Broomhall. He was delighted to tell me the good news again. The Avastin had shrunk the tumour dramatically; it was now half of its original size, 7.5 by 5 centimetres, which when looked at three dimensionally, is smaller still. The operation would be carried out by two teams of surgeons; first the bowel surgeon, Mr Bradley would remove my entire ascending colon along with the appendix and gall bladder as they are of no use and this would be followed by the liver surgeon who would remove the entire left liver lobe. It was unusual to have both operations in one but Mr Broomhall was happy to do this for me. He did advise, however, that it is often the case that only after cutting open would he know if the removal of the tumour was possible. If it was not possible to remove it with clearance of good cells, he would have to just stitch me up again. I understood all the risks and he asked me what I wanted to do. I laughed as this is what I had been aiming for over the whole year. This is what I wanted so much: a 30% chance of a cure if the operation was successful!

During this pre-op appointment with Mr Broomhall, he went through all my options; he laughed again when he saw my eagerness to have the operation. There was one bit of bad news that I now learned about. A scar had been noticed on my right lung and he wanted me to have a detailed scan of this after the operation. If it was cancer, he told me that he would cut it out. Obviously, this was a set back. We all appreciated what this meant if the cancer had spread at this point but we had to move forward and remain positive; you could only take one step at a time but it made matters so much harder.

11 *Preparing for the Op*

Mum came down and arranged to stay with a friend near Bromsgrove. She did not want to get in the way or be a trouble to Mark when I was in hospital and she also wanted to be able to stay with me when I was there, just to be there. Poor Mum planned to travel in by train and then get the shuttle service bus to the hospital. It would be quite a trek for her at her age as she was 86 and it would also be dark because of the time of year. Still, she wanted to do this.

I had to go to the hospital the day before the operation. I had read up as much as I could about what to expect and tried to warn Mum about the many tubes that would be attached to me so that she wouldn't be too shocked. I did feel a bit apprehensive but I also felt excited. I was being given such a chance. What a change from that day when I was told there was no hope.

My bed wasn't ready and the three of us sat in the day room for quite some time. I left my bags with the nurses and we talked for a bit but it was difficult to really have a conversation. I told Mark and Mum not to worry and thanked them for everything they had done. I was due to have my operation in the morning of the next day unless there was an emergency. An emergency before me could only be the case if there was to be a liver transplant because there had been a donor. My operation was deemed to be of importance because it involved two teams of surgeons at the same time and obviously, they had to be available.

After a while I told Mark to go home as I would be fine and it was pointless for him to wait; I knew what was to happen and only had to be given my bed. Mark was going to take Mum to stay with Mary and I could see that she was reluctant to leave me alone. There was another Asian man in the day room with his two children and it was good to listen to the energy of the little ones as they jumped on the chairs. Mum told me how brave I was and gave me a big hug as she kissed me goodbye and Mark told me how much he loved me. This was the difficult bit as we all knew what we were thinking. The television was on and I directed my eyes towards it as I sat there but tears trickled down my face; the kind man asked me if I was all right and I assured him that I was. It wasn't too long before I was called to my bed and went through some form filling. I spoke to the anaesthetist and signed the consent forms; later I was brought the gowns and surgical stockings I would be putting on for the operation. I was timetabled to be the first into the theatre the next day, about 6am in the morning. Yes, this was all really happening. I went to take a shower so that I would be clean.

12 *Happy to Die in Order to Live*

I did my best to sleep that night but a strange bed, a strange place and all that was to happen, kept me awake. I kept asking the nurse if I was definitely first and she checked for me. Yes, I was first. I was in my gown and waiting early in the morning. Mark had phoned me and everyone was anxious. Dr Farrago had said, 'It's one thing to get to the operation, it's another to get out of it'. I had had it explained what a major operation this was. We all understood the risks.

You can imagine the feeling when I was suddenly told that there had been a donor and there was to be a liver transplant before me. It was now questionable whether I would have my operation that day at all. I was pleased for the person on the receiving end but it did not make my situation any easier. A transplant would take at least five hours. I phoned Mark and he came straight up to the hospital to be with me. Time did pass and all we had to do was wait. Mr Broomhall and his team worked all this time during which I had some more visits from Mr Bradley, who was standing by, and went through the part of the operation he would perform. I also had a visit from a member of the research team who asked me if I would donate the healthy part of my liver when it had been removed. He said that it was difficult to obtain healthy liver for testing new drugs. After a few hours, I told Mark to go home for lunch but promised to keep him informed.

Suddenly, I was told that I was going into theatre; it was about twelve thirty; Mr Broomhall had been working intensively for six hours and now he was going to operate on me straight after. What an incredible man! I phoned Mark immediately but I had to be quick and we gave each other all our love. This happened so fast and before I knew it, I was in the room with the anaesthetists. I felt incredibly calm; I was quite happy as I had complete trust in these incredibly clever people. If it wasn't for their hard work I wouldn't have a chance. I had told Mark and Mum not to come over that day as I would probably be asleep; to be honest, I didn't know what I would be. This certainly was a time when you gather your thoughts about everything you have and make the best decision. I knew that this may be the end as the anaesthetic went through my vein but I was so content; I felt so lucky.

I must have been smiling as I went into theatre. The next thing I knew, I was being awakened. My first sensation was that I was still alive. Then the next fleeting thought was, 'Is it all done? Did they take out both the tumours?'

'Yes, it's all fine,' I was assured. 'They were able to remove both of them.'

I felt OK and it seemed like only seconds before they were wheeling me out of recovery and through the corridor. As I was taken through the door, sitting there were Mark and Mum who jumped up. They had come over and sat there all the time. Mark said that he couldn't possibly sit waiting at home and when he phoned Mum to ask if she wanted to come, she was only too ready. The operation had taken five hours; what a wait that must have been for them. Mr Broomhall was on his mobile as he came through the door. Still full of spirit, he cut off his conversation to speak to Mark. 'What a woman,' he said. 'She's the only person who's smiled all the way through the operation!' That smile on my face during anaesthetic must have stayed there through my sleep. Mark asked Simon Broomhall if the operation was a success and he said that he was able to take out the complete tumour; he was very happy but we would have to wait for the results of the biopsy on the surrounding tissue which would take a few days. I could sense the feeling of relief. Mark told me how much he loved me and Mum told me how brave I was. I felt that I was just there; it was everyone else who had to be brave.

I was given a bed at the end of the High Dependency Ward, a long ward with about a dozen beds and with a nurse allocated to every two patients. I had been in the ward before as I asked to see it when I had my appointment with Mr Broomhall the week before. It all helps when you are familiar with your surroundings. Mark and Mum sat by me and I was surprised at how alert I actually was. I felt drowsy but not sick; the adrenaline must have been gushing at the thought of what had been achieved for me. I had all the tubes they told me about: one really thick one into the base of my neck with several little tubes stemming into that in case I needed a transfusion during the op; one thick one to drain away fluid; one from the liver to collect bile which looked disgusting and smelt foul and a catheter as I would not be able to get out of bed for a while. I had an oxygen mask which I used generously; it really helped and I was attached to an epidural with the related tubes as well. There was a large white bandage over my operation cut which stretched from halfway down my right side right across my entire front under my chest.

Mark and Mum gave me all their love and prayers and said such beautiful things. I felt so content, so at peace, so happy.

13 *Lucy in the Sky, with Diamonds!*

I was at one end of the ward and I became aware of a lady in the next bed who seemed to be making some very important phone calls. It seemed strange to be doing this in an intensive care ward; one call after another after another! I soon realised that she was imagining all these people at the other end of the line, which was amusing at first but soon became irritating. She never spoke to me or even looked across and I wondered whether the drug she was taking was affecting her. She carried this on all morning. Feeling on edge, I was becoming more aware of myself; it was difficult to turn and my stomach was swelling. I had a wonderful nurse to attend to me whose name was Lydia. My stomach continued to swell and was getting really uncomfortable. I had an epidural to relieve this but I was very much in pain with the swelling. Lydia asked me how uncomfortable I was on a scale of one to ten and I said seven. She brought some spray to test the effectiveness of the epidural and sprayed a little of this in several places. Around the cut I could feel it freeze and down my left leg it didn't seem so cold.

'Oh my God!' she exclaimed. 'She has no pain relief and only complaining of a seven!' The anaesthetist was called from theatre and said that the epidural wasn't working. She proposed to give me morphine that I could control myself. My stomach continued to swell and I felt that I was going to burst. I could not bear this and thought of those six men who were on the news not that long ago; they were students on a trial drug that went badly wrong and they swelled up so suddenly that all their buttons popped off and they were in danger of dying. I now knew what they felt like. The doctor told me that it would take a while for my bowels to work and for the air to escape. At the moment it was expanding inside me.

It wasn't long before I was fitted with the morphine machine; I lay pretty helpless just pressing this button. It wasn't possible to overdose but on checking, it appeared that I was using up to my limit! In this doped state, I could hear talk about a patient in the opposite bed to the right who supposedly had MRSA. My brain was alerted to this conversation; strange things were going on. This lady was then moved to the opposite end of the ward and the entire area around this bed was cleaned. I heard the nurses talking about the porter who had wheeled her to the ward; he would have to be contacted and tested for the bug. I couldn't believe my ears but knew that I wasn't imagining this, even though I was doped. Two patients were being moved to other wards after complaining; I wanted to go as well. I remember thinking that Mark would be furious if he knew.

I called Lydia over and quietly asked her about the situation; she confirmed that the aforementioned woman had MRSA but there was very little risk as the medical staff were very careful and used the cleansing gel before attending each patient. I wasn't comfortable about this and in a high dependency ward as well! That woman should be in isolation! I was mulling this over in my mind when a doctor came into the ward. I told him about my fears quietly and he said that he fully understood; he said that he would feel the same and he appreciated the fact that I had spoken to him quietly. He tried to reassure me that the nurses would be very careful and cleanse their hands but I had noticed that they were not all doing this and told him so. He promised to speak to them to ensure this would be done systematically.

The night must have passed with me dozing and waking. The lovely day nurses had gone home and there were several nurses on duty from the agency. They spent much of their time huddled together, chatting at the far end of the ward; not checking the screens full of data behind each patient. Everyone is human, and nursing is not a job I could do. Things quietened down later and, even though the morphine made you drowsy, it also had the power to alert your senses to a high degree. However, it made you hallucinate and I had some awful visions at times: flying and whirling. Who would ever want to take drugs voluntarily?

My stomach was now tight and hard and pulled against my cut. I couldn't even turn sideways and was frightened that the cut would pull apart. The first doctor who examined me spoke about putting a drain to my stomach through my nose and I winced. It was normal for the bowel to take time to work. I took the opportunity of speaking about the MRSA patient and he was quite abrupt in response, saying that one third of patients had MRSA in the hospital and there was no risk as long as the cleanser was used. He added that the woman was now cleared of it and confirmed this with the nurses. I still did not feel happy as I knew that my cut would have to be redressed that day and so I asked to be moved out of the ward.

What a terrible day that was! Lydia came back on duty which was comforting but she was rushed to a lady who had been stretchered into the far end of the ward near the doctors' station. She tried to resuscitate the lady and begged her to open her mouth as she sprayed something into it. The woman was absolutely screaming at each spray and must have refused to do any more in the end. The screaming continued and continued until everything went suddenly and completely silent. I was in the middle of saying something out loud and on hearing my voice, stopped in mid flow. I heard my one word against the silence and knew what had happened. Lydia walked with her head down slowly out of the ward. I called her quietly as she walked past me and told her I was sorry. 'It's part of my job,' she replied kindly. 'You get used to it.'

It wasn't long after this that a very loud banging of metal started. There was a store room just outside the ward; I could see it from my bed. Two workmen had turned up and were fitting metal shelves together by banging them into place. The entire little room had to be fitted out with these shelves. After about an hour, Lydia went into the room and must have said something; she tried to close the door which helped but it was soon left open again with people looking in and out and more shelves arriving. It really was absolutely dreadful and the lady opposite me complained several times as she was right next to it. Nothing could be done as these shelves had to be fitted. This didn't help my discomfort and I was only eased by pressing on my morphine button more and more. The woman next to me continued to make her important phone calls. Goodness knows what state I was in when Mark and Mum came to see me. They were wonderful and kind and listened to all I had to say; Mark spoke of Jevan and Aidan who always sent their love and I knew their thoughts were with me. From a stage where I thought it impossible for my stomach to tighten any more, it got bigger and harder. There was still talk about a drain into it and I winced again.

Lydia changed shifts in the evening and a male nurse called Michael was given responsibility for me. I slept so soundly that the night did not even seem to have existed and in the morning, I told one of the nurses how wonderful it had been. 'It hasn't been quiet for us!' she exclaimed and I did not understand the significance of her statement until later on. Michael had barely introduced himself when he returned to tell me that I was being moved out of the ward. As I was wheeled away in my bed, the lady in the opposite bed spoke out,

'It shouldn't be you,' she said loudly. 'It should be the other woman. I hope that I'm next to you when I come out of this ward.' I must have created havoc during the night, but what had I done? I was quite happy to be moving out and was now in a room with six beds. It was very, very warm and this made it more uncomfortable for me than I already was. At least now, when my cut was redressed, it wouldn't be in a ward with MRSA but I wondered what I had said to have influenced this sudden move. Had I said something in my sleep or under the morphine? These drugs were making me hallucinate every time I closed my eyes. I asked one of the nurses, who was friendly to me, what had happened, but she feigned ignorance and laughed. I was quite embarrassed and didn't know what I had done. And to this day, I still don't know!

14 *Christit! You Know it ain't Easy*

That morning, my cut was redressed. I could see what had been done; about 50 staples held the cut in place, so neatly done it was tremendous. I learned that different surgeons used different methods to join the cut; some used strong sticky tape, others stitched it up and Mr Broomhall used staples that would be removed at a later date after I returned home.

I had visits from Aidan who was at university in Birmingham but he had to walk such a long way and wasn't very well himself. Mum and Mark came every day to see me and Jevan came with them on some occasions. John and Eirian came over from Ledbury and Margaret came bringing Mum with her. Mum was staying with her friend, Mary, and had such a difficult trek on the train and then she had to get the shuttle bus at the hospital. It was October and got dark very early and I was so concerned for her.

My stomach had grown so much; I was only allowed to sip a few drops of water per half day and I felt I could demolish a litre of it. That night was probably my worst; the first night in the new ward. My stomach must have reached its bursting point and I started to be sick; I pressed the buzzer for the nurse and kept pressing it. I held my mouth closed and tried to signal for a sick bowl. The message got through at last with my urgent gestures. I was so sick; it seemed to go on forever and I filled at least six sick bowls. I couldn't speak but there were about four nurses tending to me now. I must have woken the entire ward and there was nothing I could do about it; I was completely exhausted.

The nurses were nothing like the dedicated nurses in the high dependency unit; some were lovely and helpful, always rushing around and doing what they could; unfortunately, there were several who set out to do as little as possible, taking half an hour to walk across the ward and never coming to your aid when you pressed the buzzer. It was so frustrating, being stuck in the bed and not able to do the slightest thing yourself. It was even more frustrating when the nurse would move the bed table aside to take your temperature and forgot to return it so it was out of reach.

The doctor saw me in the morning and said he had advised me to have my stomach drained. Unfortunately it was 'slow nurse' who was given the job to do this. My throat was already sore after the operation and I had to have a tube put through my nose; I was told to swallow to help it to go down and it was pushed down in stages. It was, I must say, dreadful. The tube was then stuck to my nose and a bag was attached to the end of this, yet another collection bag along with the operation drain, the bile and the catheter. Slow nurse couldn't find the correct tape to do the nose attachment so she used some ordinary stuff. All this was quite traumatic but when the stomach was pumped out, it was such an instant relief. More and more horrid browny yellow fluid kept coming out and this was all measured and noted. I gave a deep sigh when she finished; it was worth all the pain.

Mark came to see me later that morning and I told him about all my adventures. I was allowed to slide off the bed onto the seat and he helped me to change my nightdress which was stained, sweaty and smelly. Alas, on removing this, it also removed my stomach tube which slid out because the wrong tape had been used and the tube had become unstuck from my nose. I just could not believe it as I saw the end of the tube loose in my hand. I called slow nurse and what did she do? She laughed and said it would have to be done again. Have to be done again? Not all that again! I wanted to cry! Another efficient nurse did the job this time but it was the same procedure. My throat was so sore I could hardly take my tablets, even after breaking them into morsels. It was very difficult to talk but I made the effort. At least now I was not going to burst.

Time did heal and my throat slowly got better from day to day. I felt so sorry for Mark and Mum who came daily to see me; parking was such a problem there. I felt sorry for Aidan trying to fit in visits between lectures. However, I was improving but for a slight temperature which was causing concern. I was put on an antibiotic drip to cure this but it was later decided unnecessary and removed. The ward was so hot that Mark brought our own fan from home which was a real relief. I was not supposed to use it till it was safety checked but this was quietly overlooked by the staff as it was a help to everyone.

I don't usually complain but, in this ward, no-one had any time for you as they were so short staffed. I was encouraged to sit on a chair for a while each morning and on one morning, my catheter didn't work and leaked, creating a puddle on the floor. I had to call the nurse who was obviously busy as they always were. No-one cleaned up the urine and it dried below my feet, only to be cleaned the next day during the usual cleaning rounds. I was so pleased when the doctor said that the catheter could be removed and I could now use the toilet with help. One night, I felt the need to go to the toilet as nothing solid had as yet passed through me. The nurse brought a bed pan! There was no chance of any success on this, lying flat on my back, uncomfortable!

After a few days of getting more and more smelly and feeling very conscious of the acrid stink from the bile drip that my visitors had to endure, I asked for a shower. Four days after the operation, I was now moving about a little. I had my shower on my own and it was quite an unnerving experience. There were only two bathrooms in the whole unit and there was always a queue for the newer one. You couldn't use the loo without someone trying the door handle, so you were always trying to be quick. I therefore decided to use the older toilets which had a stand-up shower in them. I carefully worked my way around the piles of bedpans and sick bowls piled around the corners of the small space as this room was also used as a storeroom for these. Stepping carefully into the shower and leaving my crutches on the side, I managed to wash. It was really wonderful to rub away the smells and feel the water on me. It was not easy to move and water had built up to four inches in the tray so I decided to try stepping out and drying myself. All this I managed and felt quite exhausted but when I attempted to slide the door open, I discovered it was stuck tight. It was a rickety wooden door and it refused to slide along its channel. I looked for a help cord but could not find one; I was later shown that it hung along the corner of the shower but it was difficult to see as it disappeared into a groove. I heard voices along the corridor outside and banged and shouted at the top of my voice. 'I can hear someone shouting,' I heard the nurse say so I shouted louder, saying that I was stuck in the shower room. It was a jolly nurse who came to my rescue and saw me back to my bed. I felt that I had had quite some exercise that day but I was pleased that I had now washed.

Food was another issue. I wasn't allowed any food and only

allowed to sip a little more water as the days went by and it was an ordeal to see all the trays of food being brought to everyone else but me along with the orders for the next day. My temperature was still a little raised and so the prospect of being allowed food was drifting further and further away; along with this, the target time for going home was disappearing. The possibility of returning to humanity on the ninth day came and went and it was now the weekend with less chance of anything being decided. On the tenth day, I was surprised when the doctor said that I could eat a little and I looked forward to food time eagerly. The food always looked and smelt good and after all this time in the hospital, this was to be my first meal there. Disappointed at being ignored as the trays were distributed, I asked for something to eat. I had not been able to order my food on the previous day and this appeared to have posed a problem. The nurse was running around and out of breath and in the middle of a run, asked me what I would like. I thought that I had better be sensible so I replied, 'Some soup and bread roll would be nice and some ice cream please'. She ran around looking for some that had not been claimed and brought me back some half-eaten cold soup which she virtually dropped in front of me. She then ran off to get a slice of bread out of their fridge and disappeared even before I had time to tell her that I had not been given a spoon. What a disappointing first meal; even the ice cream was melted. No spoon, cold soup and warm ice cream. What a shambles!

On the eleventh day I was allowed to go home. What bliss!

15 *I Believe in Miracles*

Returning home was so wonderful. I remembered the thoughts that had gone through my mind before leaving and here I was, ready for recovery and having been given the chance of a cure. I was seated down and fussed over and Mark insisted on bringing down the bed settee and a blanket for me to stretch out on which Jevan helped him to do. Mum was relieved that I had a bed to lie on, never wanting to interfere on any matter. The furniture was re-arranged but it all seemed to be very tidy and not in an upturn as I expected it to be. I stretched out on what was to be my place for many days to come. It really was comfortable and I was there in company and in the middle of all the action! The house looked lovely and I had been sent beautiful flowers and gifts from so many people. The cards never stopped coming and I was given all the encouragement one could get. Mum prayed all the time, said 'The Novena' and so did many of our relations and her friends from all over the world. I couldn't be given a stronger chance; a miracle was being prayed for.

Mum used her expert skills to make the tastiest curries, keeping them mild for me. I was able to eat a little and it was so enjoyable. It was also lovely to have the television there and to be able to doze off when I wanted. Everyone worked around me, keeping the noise down when my eyes were closed and tending to my every need.

I did have a lot of pain but I kept taking the morphine and I expected to have discomfort after what had been done. I had some fluid around the lung which made breathing and yawning quite difficult so it would take two goes to have a yawn. I got to know all the District Nurses very well; they were all lovely and redressed the wound, took blood tests and checked my wellbeing.

Within a few days of my return, the scan was booked back in Birmingham to check the scar on my right lung. This was arranged and carried out very efficiently and a few days after that, I was told that this scar had not developed further; it could have occurred many years ago from an attack of bronchitis I suffered in my twenties. This was fantastic news! Now I could move on again! Mum was with me when my GP gave me this news and we both cried with joy. This was truly amazing!

At this stage, I was thinking of reapplying to the PCT to fund my Avastin post-operatively. They could see that the drug had worked for me as it had shrunk my tumour sufficiently to enable the operation. I had to prove to them that I was an 'exceptional' patient for funding to be granted. I contacted Bowel Cancer UK to help me to word my letter. My sister-in-law, Eirian, had told me that she had heard about a lady on the news who needed Avastin and this charity had helped them. I phoned them and a very helpful woman listened to my story and went through what I should write. After I had written the letter, she listened while I read it back to her and approved it. I sent this off, hoping for a positive response. I didn't realise at the time what publicity this was to give rise to, nationally, and I will write a lot more about this as my story progresses.

16 *They're Gonna Crucify Me!*

After a few days, Mark returned to work on shortened time. However, it wasn't long after this that I experienced a severe headache and shivers. Mum was resting downstairs with me and I didn't want to worry or disturb her. I lay as still as I could to help the pain that was getting increasingly uncomfortable, knowing that Mark would be home quite soon. When Mark returned and suggested ringing the doctor, I readily agreed as I was now feeling faint and dizzy. Dr Alden arrived within minutes and checked my temperature and lungs. I had got a very high temperature and he wanted to call an ambulance to take me directly to hospital. We were fortunate in that the hospital is just around the corner and Mark said that he was quite happy to drive me there as this would be quicker.

He helped me out of the car and wheeled me around to the ward labelled MAU, as directed. This was the Medical Assessment Unit and we were asked to go to register in the outpatient clinic to have the usual checks done there as it was busy in the ward. We went there and waited for hours with very little done. I was eventually taken into a side room for blood tests, given an x-ray in the relevant department and then a charming female doctor asked me several questions about my medical history, filling in the forms for me. A doctor was to see me before I was sent to the ward. However, it had got so late, and although I was allowed to wait in the side room where I could lie down, clinic was now closing. Mark and I were given a sandwich by a very helpful, cheerful nurse.

I now had to be transferred to a trolley bed in a corridor of the MAU. There were about six beds alongside each other and here we waited for another length of time. It was like a circus with such a noise and chaos around. On my left was an old man who had got himself out of his trolley bed and was walking around half naked. He had wet all over the floor before someone came to help him to a toilet. On my right was a large Russian woman. She had a number of family members around her and they were talking very loudly in Russian and taking up all my space to the right; it was uncomfortable in the circumstances.

Eventually, a doctor in a surgeon's green outfit came to me and checked my lungs. He told me I had water in the right lung, which I knew, and this was the problem. He would have to remove it by pushing a tube through my back to reach the lung and syringe out the water. There was no anaesthetic and I did not like the idea but I had no choice. Mark was with me and helped so much. I had to sit on the edge of the bed and lean on the bedside table with my arms folded. This was the most painful thing I have had done and tears were pouring from my eyes. The worst news was that it had not been successful and had to be done again. The doctor repeated the procedure but again, it was unsuccessful and he said that he could not do it again. I was relieved and I wondered why this had to be done in a corridor and who this doctor was. Around midnight, I was taken to a bed in MSSU, or Medical Short Stay Unit in a bay of four and felt much happier. I was to stay in hospital for a while.

The next morning, I was seen by a consultant who told me that no more needles would be pushed into my back and he put me on a strong general antibiotic that was administered intravenously. Although my headaches persisted, I did feel better before long. Tests were taken to determine what infection I may have; some of these tests would take quite a few days for results to show. Swabs were taken for MRSA and various other blood tests. I was told that I may have developed an abscess in my liver or that the cancer may have come back. I was quite worried so Mum immediately went over to the Rowan Suite as it was a Tuesday and hoped to talk to Dr Farrago as this was the day he held his clinic. With her luck or her prayers, she managed to meet Dr Farrago in the corridor and told him about my condition. He promised to come over to see me and discuss my situation with the doctors in the ward.

Dr Farrago kept to his word as he has always done. He showed sympathy and did remind me of the risks involved in my treatment. 'Could the cancer have come back so soon?' I asked him. 'Is it possible?'

'If it has, we have done all we can do,' was his answer and he was, of course, right.

I felt much happier that he had come over and he kept a track on my progress from that point. Tests showed that I had an abscess in my liver and The Queen Elizabeth admitted that it would have been infected during the operation, the bowel being operated on straight after the liver, as the infection was e-coli from the colon. It was a relief that nothing was indicating that the cancer had returned; my antibiotic was changed to match the bug it was treating and an ultrasound scan was planned during which a tube would be pushed directly into the abscess to drain it. I was quite nervous at the thought of all this.

'Will I have an anaesthetic?' I asked the doctor.

'Yes, you will have a local anaesthetic, an injection,' the reply came reassuringly. The nurses here were very caring; they could not have been more attentive and understood what I'd been through.

The scan seemed to happen sooner than I expected. I was wheeled to the x-ray department and waited among other patients for my name to be called. The nurses were wonderful and gentle in their manner and transferred me to a couch as I needed to be stretched out. Everything was done as clinically as in an operation. The consultant radiologist was about seven foot tall and sounded Austrian or Norwegian. He was very gentle too and gave me confidence as he explained everything that he did. He told me that he would give me an injection that would probably be the most painful part of the procedure; after that I must tell him if the pain got too uncomfortable. I was given a fair amount of anaesthetic in the injection. After that, the consultant pushed a thin tube through me; he was looking at the picture of my left liver lobe on the monitor and was directing the tube so that it punctured the tough wall of the abscess. This part was not painful but you could feel the tube being pushed firmly a bit at a time which felt really odd. A drain tube was then inserted through the first tube and the consultant used a syringe to extract three large syringes full of horrid yellow stuff from the abscess. This was measured and sent for analysis. On completion of all this, a drainage bag was attached to the end of the tube so that the abscess could continue to drain over the next few days. The antibiotics would now be given a better chance to take effect.

I was quite relieved when all this was over and I was back in the ward. I felt a bit sore for a day or so and had to be careful on showering, of course, with the 'handbag' attached to the end of the tube, plus another tube and stand for the antibiotic drip. The nurses were kind enough to re-dress and keep the area clean every morning and I never had to wait long for this to be done after my shower.

Although the drain was only supposed to be needed for a few days, there was still yellow stuff coming out several days after the scan. However, I had an appointment arranged for that Friday at the Queen Elizabeth in Birmingham so I was allowed home the day before and told that the drain could be removed when I went to Birmingham. The antibiotic had been changed to tablet form which allowed my return home so I got out of the car with my new 'handbag' and retook my place on the bed settee. Everyone was pleased for me to be back but, most of all, I was pleased.

17 *The Return of the Abscess*

I hardly seemed to be out of one hospital when I had to visit the next; I had my operation check-up to go to on the Friday and I was so looking forward to seeing Mr Broomhall to thank him but unfortunately, he could not be there. I saw the professor who looked just like Einstein. He was obviously highly intelligent and had that manner of scattiness that often goes with these attributes. He could not find some of my reports from the hospital regarding the analysis of the tumours. Fortunately, I had already received copies of these as Mr Broomhall's secretary had faxed them to my GP a while ago, at my request. I had a 2cm clearance of the cancer cells around the removed liver tumour and the top and bottom of the removed colon were also free of disease, so the operation had been a great success. The chemo nurse was present; she knew all the details along with how to operate the computer and I had met her on several occasions before, during and after my operation.

Anyway, I asked whether the professor would remove my drain bag and he directed me to the couch. I was quite nervous about the removal of this but it just tickled its way out at his pull.

'Gosh! That didn't hurt at all!' I exclaimed and he replied, 'I would have told you if it was going to.'

The meeting had been interrupted by someone coming in and asking the professor for something and he must have been thinking about this because, all of a sudden, he jumped up and walked off in mid sentence. The chemo nurse apologised without making an apology directly and talked to us for a while more before we left to return home.

Hopefully, this time I was returning to stay at home. I looked forward to this so much. The district nurses were able to come less frequently and were able to remove some of the dressings completely as the scars were drying up nicely. Unfortunately, within a few days, my temperature was spiking again and I had been told to contact the doctor immediately if this happened. I knew my symptoms from last time and I didn't delay. I rang the surgery and the receptionist took my details; it was late in the afternoon and surgery was near its end. The receptionist rang me back a little later and asked whether I could go up to the surgery. I contacted Mark at work and he returned home quickly to take me but we had only just started out when my mobile rang and the receptionist told me that the doctor did not need to see me; I should just monitor the situation! Perhaps she also said that the doctor would phone me later after her surgery. I told her that I was already on my way at the time so I was told that I may as well go in. I had to wait a long time in the waiting room but the doctor did see me in the end; it was a doctor who did not know me or my background, I think. She said that she could refer me to the hospital if I wanted but she did not think it necessary. Much as I loathed having to go to hospital, I did realise what was happening to me from the last time and asked to be referred directly. Mark took me straight there and, as I expected, I was kept in again. Round two; another abscess; I knew it all!

18 *To Diarrhoea or not to Diarrhoea!*

The same process was to be carried through but this time, I thought I knew what was to come. I didn't at all! I suppose that I was really fed up of being in hospital and having no privacy. I was placed in a bay of four which stank of smelly shoes. It was revolting! I asked to be moved and, to their word, the nurses did their best for me. I was taken downstairs to the basement where they dealt with strokes and infectious diseases. I was given a side room that had just been bleached to kill infectious bugs but the toilet smelt of wee and my mother-in-law splashed her perfume all over to try to help alleviate the smell. I had the same tests for MRSA and the usual blood tests and an ultrasound and drain were again arranged.

It was a different consultant this time. He gave the injection and decided to push the wire through the ribs to get the best contact with the cyst. The pain, I must say, was excruciating this time and he had to stop. He then had to repeat this in a different place from the front and duly pushed the wire through; again, the wire went through and through and each push was really painful. However, it was done and that was the important thing. He collected the horrid yellow stuff and attached the 'handbag'.

I was left in a lot of discomfort and it was difficult to move or to put weight on my foot as the pain shot up to my chest. This was made worse when I was told at 11pm that I had to be moved again that night. I stayed awake because of this and had to pack my belongings again when I was really tired. I was promised another side room but in the correct ward with the doctor I should have been under. This was my only consolation. I had, by now, been visited by several consultants and was told that I was known all over the hospital! I knew how much time was being given to me and never stopped appreciating how much care I was getting. At two in the morning, the bed was ready and I was moved; I set up all my things straight away although I was in pain and then tried to get some sleep knowing that the hospital day starts at 6.30 in the morning. To my disgust, I was told the next morning that I would have to move again. This was the bed manager who decided that I didn't need a side room and there had been an outbreak of diarrhoea. There had been a complaint in the local press about this by other patients. I told this manager that I would not move, that this was outrageous and that I was fighting for my life. I later discovered that this was indeed a very dangerous and critical time for me; I honestly didn't realise how dangerous this was at the time. The consultant and nurses all supported me and said that I should not be moved again; four times in three days was ludicrous. It was after the tests came back that it was discovered I did have a super bug, originating from the e-coli, and that I had to be isolated and that I was indeed, by chance, in the right place for isolating infectious diseases!

While I was in hospital, I had a response from the PCT written on the 5th December, 2007. Mark brought the letter in to me, full of expectation but I must admit that my hopes were not as high as Mark's to a positive response and I was right. They refused funding for my post-operative course of Avastin because they said that I could not prove it was the Avastin that had shrunk the tumour; it could have been the chemotherapy. They also said that they could not pay for the treatment I had already had because I paid for it privately! How else would I have received the treatment?

All this sounds full of complaint and troublesome; indeed it was troublesome but I had the best care you could get. On top of the medical care, Mark continued to be with me whenever he could, cooking and bringing curries in for me. Mum came back from Otley and she carried on the visits in the day when Mark returned to work and she carried in these curries, hot and ready to eat. I'm sure that she must have walked at such a pace to get to me with the food, piping hot. There was so much thought behind everything she did.

Dr Farrago has always done everything he could and he visited me again, giving his expert advice. If I was cleared of the abscess, I could still have the post-operative chemo but time was running out. This time the abscess did not take quite so long to drain and I had a second scan to check what was happening. The consultant was to remove the tube and I knew, or thought I knew, that this wouldn't hurt. It had to be done but it was quite different this time; the tube came out with a complete curl at the end and it was this that caused me so much discomfort as it was pulled out even though the doctor was as gentle as he could be. Anyway, I was on the up again and that's what mattered and soon I could go home. I would have to take the strong antibiotics for several weeks.

19 *To Quango or not to Quango!*

On returning home, one of the first things I wanted to do was to contact Bowel Cancer UK to inform them of the response from the PCT and ask their advice. They had sent me a useful pack of information that mentioned approaching your MP for support, along with contacting the local press and getting a letter from your oncologist and GP. I did all of these things and fantastic letters were written by all in my support. It was at this point that I first spoke to Ian Beaumont, Director of Communications, and he gave me all the encouragement I needed. I sent him copies of all the letters mentioned and he immediately got one of the lawyers who work on a pro bono basis to help me with my appeal against the PCT decision. This was quite a lengthy process and something of a test case; no-one had tried to make a claim retrospectively before and my new course of chemo plus Avastin had already started. This would cost another £10,500.

Meanwhile, I contacted the local press, Worcester News, who were incredibly interested in my story; I was really surprised. A reporter wanted to come around immediately but I delayed him till the next day. A photographer came and took what seemed like hundreds of photos. I had e-mailed the BBC and BBC Hereford and Worcester were on the phone, wanting a live interview. I agreed to take part in a live interview the next morning on the Breakfast

Show. I couldn't believe that other people would be so interested! So all this took place and Ian Beaumont was interviewed before me; it was quite nerve racking as I had never done anything like this before. That same day, Wednesday 9th January 2008, I was front page of the Worcester News with a large photo and headline, '21K to save my life!' This was the start of my campaigning for greater access to these new potentially life-saving drugs.

I remember that Wednesday so vividly as I went to St Richard's and there was a lot of talk about the article. People wanted to know about the details and commented on how disgusting the whole affair was. They couldn't believe that I had to pay for all the drugs that I was previously getting on the NHS because I wanted to take one extra drug recommended by my doctors. Many people had heard the broadcast on the radio that morning. Ian Beaumont was pleased with the publicity this was getting and the fact that the immoral nature of the situation was being brought out in the open.

On my return home from St. Richard's, I was tired as I had not had any afternoon rest. I switched on the answer phone as I routinely do and was shocked to have a number of messages from various press agencies, one from Birmingham, some freelance and there was also a letter hand delivered from a press agency in Bristol along with a recorded message. I decided to phone the Bristol agency since they were so keen. They offered to pay me a thousand pounds for a contract to write my story in the 'Your Life' pages of The Mirror as an exclusive. I consulted with Ian Beaumont and he soon became my advisor on everything I did for the press. He always warned me as to what to be wary of and gave the go-ahead when he envisaged no problem. I felt safe to have the strength of his wisdom on grounds that I was so inexperienced in.

Following this there were many more contacts with the press, local and national. Sometimes Ian phoned me when the Press had contacted Bowel Cancer UK for someone to do a case study on and I was always willing. There were many similar cases to mine in other counties; people were stepping forward to tell the public that, after they had paid all their taxes, they were being deprived of potentially life-saving drugs when they needed them. Across the water in Europe these were widely available and free. Britain was turning into a Third World Country as far as this was concerned. My story was printed in The Sun, The Mail, The Express and numerous local papers in the county and in Birmingham. I felt pleased with the response that Bowel Cancer UK had helped me to achieve. I felt so strongly that I had come from a situation of 'no hope' to a situation in which I now had a chance of a cure and it was Avastin that had made this possible. My hair was now falling off for the third time but I had got used to this and it wasn't important. I had met people out there who are now wondering whether their husband or wife would be alive if they had somehow paid for this drug. I could not believe that this was happening in England. Worse still, there were some authorities where the drugs were being funded and some that rejected all requests for it. It became a 'post code lottery'; if you lived in Scotland, the drug was free.

20 *To Live or not to Live!*

My appeal with the PCT was fast approaching; Leanne, the solicitor working on my behalf through Bowel Cancer UK, contacted me regularly to discuss certain points; many times in the evening, as she worked late into the night. She must have spent hours on my case and splendidly produced a seventeen page document, discussing the details with other barristers to create the strongest argument. Indeed, she could not have put forward a stronger document on my behalf. She even included the comparison with the late Victoria Otley, a woman who greatly inspired me, who took her case to court and won funding for Avastin; sadly the funding came too late.

Mark took time off work and we both dressed smartly to be present at the hearing. I put on my wig as my hair had fallen again with the treatment. Strangely enough, I didn't feel too nervous; the fact that I had so much backing helped a great deal. Ian had advised me on what grounds to present my case on medical, human and legal grounds. I had bullet pointed some notes to use and was told that I would be allowed fifteen minutes to speak.

It was Friday, March the 14th. The meeting was held in the brand new offices called 'Wildwood'; a beautiful building clad in some special wood and sited on the edge of the Worcestershire

Countryside Centre. We were politely shown into a large room with a glorious oval table around which were seated about ten people. Mark and I were led to our seats and welcomed by the Chairman who was to my left at the top end of the table. There was then the chief executive of the PCT and a couple of doctors, other accountants, personal secretaries and lastly a retired teacher who was the layperson that had to be present.

I had my three pages of bullet points, one for each category that Ian had told me to speak on and here they are:

Medical Grounds

1. I was diagnosed in Nov. '06 and given 3-5 months to live.

2. First chemo *Oxaliplatin 5FU* was ineffective. The tumour in the liver progressed to 15cm by 10cm. You could see the lump protruding from the liver.

3. The second line of chemo *Irinotican 5FU* did work but not sufficiently for resection. Dr. Farrago said that further treatment of the same was **unlikely** to shrink the tumour to the extent necessary as it did not only have to shrink; it had to shrink **away** from the portal vein, the main vein to the liver. This vein had to be left but all the other veins to the left lobe were to be cut away.

4. Dr. Farrago and Mr. Broomhall advised that the addition of Avastin, if it worked, would be their recommendation for the best chance of this happening.

5. After only three of the four treatments, a scan showed that this regime shrank the tumour by 25% of its original size. It made the operation possible.

6. I am Dr. Farrago's **only** patient in his 7 years who has regressed after 1st line chemo and gone on to have a resection.

7. Avastin has given me 30-40% chance of 5 years+ survival. This has changed my position from palliative care to a chance of a **cure**.

8. Knowing its success and effectiveness on me, Dr. Farrago and Mr. Broomhall said that my best chance was to have the same regime after the op. With other cancers, this has been shown to increase survival by a further 10%.

9. Until this drug is used more in this country, statistics will not be there. In my position, I must follow my doctors' advice. Wouldn't you want that for someone you loved?

10. My doctors have told me, all of them, that if I was not exceptional, then nobody was.

Human Grounds

1. I don't give up as a person. Throughout my life-threatening illness, I have been as active as possible at each stage. I had hope, supported by my family. My Mum came down from Yorkshire to stay and I live with my husband and two successful sons.

2. Indeed, I brought my sons up as a single parent, worked full time as a teacher, never had any financial help from my ex-husband, and never claimed a single penny off the State in the 6 years on my own. The children were 6 and 7 years old then. I have paid all my taxes and am now asking for aid to save my life.

3. I have not taken a single day off work for this particular

illness, which I am told I have had for several years. I had to retire prematurely when diagnosed but I loved my job.

4. My pupils' exam results were exceptional. **Every** school I have done any work in has offered me a full time post without my applying for one. I have given up my time freely to teach pupils at lunchtimes so that they could sit two GCSEs in English and Literature instead of one.

5. At one school, the lowest set, thought to gain grades C and D, resulted with a third of them gaining grade A, a third B and a third C in their Shakespeare exam. I have motivated others to work by my enthusiasm and love of the job.

6. I have regularly attended St. Richard's Hospice as a day patient and note the PCT's involvement, recently funding five new beds. I can see their understanding towards terminally ill patients and know resources are limited. I have seen so many friends die of a lesser disease than myself. I do see my case as warranting support.

7. Whilst I accepted death, I never gave up the desire to live and always thought positively, hence doing everything possible to make me live. Adding Avastin was a major part of this.

8. If every medical possibility was not tried, I would not be here now and there would always have been a feeling of guilt left on my husband.

Legal Grounds

1. If Avastin works, it works well and results show up quickly. I was not prescribed 16 doses as stated by NICE, but 4. After

all the money already spent on me, this was a relatively small amount to aid my survival, **and it worked!**

2. The drug has not only prolonged my life, it has given me the chance of a cure.

3. I feel very grieved that a sick person has to **battle** this situation, not knowing where the money is coming from. On previous occasions, presenting my request for funding, I had only just had a major operation and before that, extensive chemotherapy.

4. My exceptionality has to be seen in the way my body tolerated 1 yr. of continuous chemotherapy and radiotherapy.

5. I refer to the letters of Dr. Carmen, Farrago and Mr. Broomhall in which they all write about my exceptionality. Surely we are going to trust our medical experts.

6. I had to make decisions re. treatment quickly. I couldn't wait for the PCT's decisions to make the appointments and so on. Wouldn't you?

7. I have the backing of Bowel Cancer UK, my oncologist, my surgeon and MP. I feel so strongly about this matter that I am prepared to follow it through to judicial review and litigation.

Thank you for listening to me.

The chairman welcomed me and his first words were obviously said to try to put me at ease. 'We're on your side,' he said. I thought about this for a time afterwards. Did he mean that they were going to agree to pay for the Avastin?

I spoke easily on the first section, 'Medical Grounds' at quite some length. On completion of this, the chairman smiled and thanked me and presumed to resume the discussion.

'I haven't finished yet!' I interrupted at which the panel all laughed. I continued and spoke for a total of about half an hour at which I was pleased. Just imagine, though, I was a person on chemotherapy, having to do this in order to plead for drugs that could save me and these were drugs recommended by my doctor. What about the people who were not able to face a panel such as this or people who were too ill to do it?

At the end, I was told that there had obviously got to be a discussion amongst themselves and that I would be notified of the decision in writing within a few days. I asked for a copy of the notes and it was agreed that this be sent to me.

I awaited the promised deadline for the decision. The postman came and went but no letter. I phoned the secretary and she swore that she had posted the letter herself; she was not allowed to tell me its contents but she would email a copy of it to me.

I did have some hope that this time I might be lucky. However, on receiving the letter, it seemed that they had not taken any notice of my barrister's weighty document and that their decision was predetermined. I had wasted my time attending the hearing but at least I had the satisfaction of looking these people making the decisions in the eye. They said that they could not pay because I had paid for the treatment privately. How else could I have had it? They also said that I could not prove it was the Avastin that had shrunk the tumour; they had taken no notice of what the top consultants had said. This decision had been made by accountants who were only looking at the money. The original letter from the PCT did arrive a week later as a slip dropped through the door; I had to collect it from the Sorting Office as the postage was underpaid!

The press were all waiting for the decision and I remember Howard Bentham of BBC Hereford and Worcester saying to me, 'Barbara, they're telling you you're not worth it!' Ian Beaumont from Bowel Cancer UK was forever helping me and he spoke again on the radio show before me. There were several articles on the internet, even on official health sites. There were more articles in the papers and the national press were getting more interested as well. I had a call from one of the producers of the 'Richard and Judy Show' on the television who interviewed me with a possibility of appearing on this show. I had just come back from chemotherapy when this happened and I remember not feeling at my best. I could not go up to London the next day and the whole thing did not materialise in the end, which was probably for the best.

I was approached by the BBC to appear on The One Show. They were featuring an article on wastage of money caused by unused repeat prescription drugs. They wanted me to tell my story of how the NHS did not have the money for people like me and people who hoard drugs could help the situation. This was filmed at home which did made it easier and Ian came down to support me, saying that he also wanted to meet me; I felt really honoured by this as he had to travel from London and it would take up his whole day. It all went well and again, family and friends eagerly watched the programme, teasing me about getting my autograph!

21 *The End of a Line and a New Beginning in France*

I was so much looking forward to the end of my chemo; could this be the end of chemo forever? I still felt grateful and thanked God for every day. You certainly don't take anything for granted when you experience something like this. Having got through to this stage, I was now given a 30 percent chance of living five years which is how the statistics are calculated.

Mark and I were making big plans for the future; we didn't want to waste time and thought about what we might really like to do. We loved France and had not been there for such a long time; indeed, I never thought I would ever see it again. What we had seen other people do in their retirement was to take their caravan and just go as they pleased, staying in one place till they wanted to move on. We would like to do that but with our long caravan and our love of luxury, we chose 4-star sites wherever possible and would have to plan so this would take time. We decided to go somewhere locally meanwhile and in February, chose a very pretty site called Beaconsfield Farm in Shrewsbury for five days. We enjoyed this trip thoroughly but it was very cold at night, minus four, and there were some problems with the electricity on the site, so the heater went off on a number of occasions. The proprietor wasn't particularly helpful either as

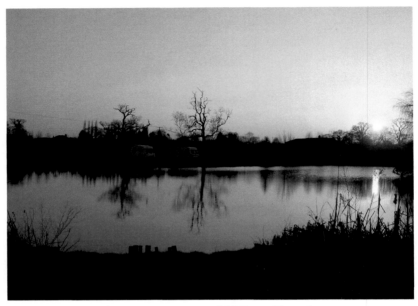

February 2008, Beaconsfield Farm, Shrewsbury

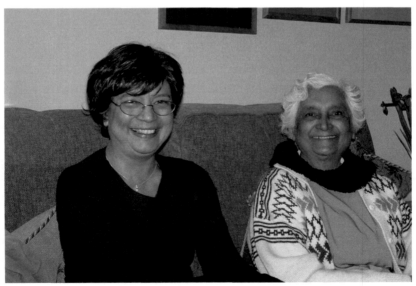

My Mum to the right at John and Eirian's house on Mother's Day

lambing had been early that year and everyone seemed to be involved in that. Anyway it was eventually sorted and we were warm again.

I would have my appointment with Dr Farrago in April and if all was well, we would be able to go away four weeks after the last chemo, following his advice, to give my body a chance to be clear of the toxic drugs before leaving the country for so long. We celebrated a lovely Mother's Day in March and Jevan and Aidan came over with beautiful flowers and cards; they were so loving and I have always felt so proud of them. Mum came down again and we all went to John and Eirian's for lunch, picking up my sister, Margaret, on the way.

There was still a long time to go before the end of my chemo so Mark and I planned a trip to France at Easter; we were going to go by Eurotunnel to stay in a chalet at a place called Licques, situated between Calais and Boulogne. We arranged all this very quickly, but made sure we took all the medication and hospital contacts. I wrote out a description of my condition and treatment in French so that Mark could present it to a doctor if I fell ill. I could not believe that I was actually going to France again; I was so excited that I forgot about my fear of tunnels and had no problem at all with the crossing.

There was a group of chalets on the campsite and we got to know the proprietors very well as it was quiet. It was wonderful to see all the fresh produce in the supermarkets again and the wonderful fish counters strewn with prawns and other seafood. Being able to do things like this made me reflect so often how fortunate I was to still be alive. We enjoyed all sorts of weather during those eight days, including thick snow which fell over two hours one afternoon!

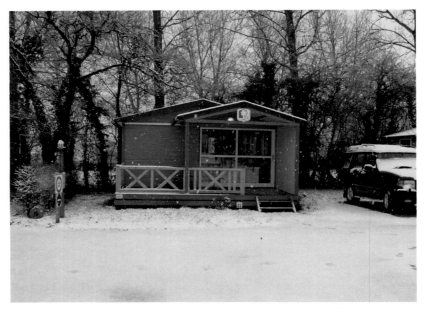

The chalet at 'Les Trois Pommiers', Licques. Easter 2008

This trip really whetted our appetite to prepare for our 'trip of a lifetime'. Mark and I talked endlessly of our plans which would last four months and hoped that Jevan and Aidan could be involved in coming out to meet us and stay for a while at some point. We looked at various routes. What we wanted was to go down the east of France, stopping south of Paris at Fontainbleau; to the Beaune region; travel south to the Mediterranean and the Camargue; across to Provence; Carcassonne; a special trip to the grotto of Lourdes; then further on to the Atlantic coast; back to the Dordogne in time for our wedding anniversary, a place we stayed at on our honeymoon; further on to mid France and then to the Loire, a campsite we visited many years ago when Jevan and Aidan were quite young and we all enjoyed. Finally, we would have six days in Normandy before our return. We avoided distances of much more than a hundred miles for each journey. We planned to travel fairly quickly to the south but have breaks on the way and we concentrated our longer stays in the places we really wanted to be in most; that way it would not be too tiring. Although no booking was required for the beginning and end of our trip, planned to start on Sunday 18th May and finish on Sunday 14th September, the middle period would cover peak holiday season and we would have to book in order to be sure of getting what we wanted. We liked a pitch with running water and drainage to connect to and these were generally found on 4-star sites. On phoning around, I discovered that there were a number of places that could not cater for a long caravan at all so every site had to be checked. I made numerous calls to France as we had to change our choices several times and finally, a plan was made, printed and deposits paid. We became members of a few select organisations which would give us discounts at certain campsites: Les Castels, ACSI and Camping Cheque and we transferred a sum of money into our French bank account. I printed out all the routes even though we bought a sat-nav for Europe. We were completely ready.

My appointment with Dr Farrago went fine; he was so pleased with my progress. All the test results were good; the CEA which indicated tumour activity by measuring protein in the blood had gone up to 3.2 but this was still well within the normal acceptance of 5. We spoke about the holiday and he told us to enjoy it. Dr Farrago was a firm believer of not wasting time although he would not knowingly let you be at risk.

Everyone was talking about our holiday and wishing us well; even though we were so organised, it did not feel real. Could this really be happening? There were a few more formalities; I had a routine appointment with Mr Broomhall at the Queen Elizabeth and Mark had to give in his notice as he was not allowed four

FROM	TO	CAMPSITE	CLUB	WATER	DATE FROM	DATE TO	HOW LONG	STAR	MOTORWAY	MILES	TOLLS	COST p.n.	TOTAL COST	DEPOSIT
1. Caen	Fontainebleau 0160704605	Courtilles du Lido 77250 Veneux les sablons	SS 43		Su 18 May	M 19 May	1	3	182	200	13	16.5	16.5€ k20€	
2. Fontainebleau B Hol	Gigny-sur-Saone 0385941690	L'Eperviere 71240	C Ch 193 CC51		M 19 May	Su 25 May	6	4	166	192	18	£10.30	£61.80	Gold card C Ch
3. Gigny-sur-Saone BHol	Valence 0475841970	Le Soleil Fruite Big pitch 6amp 26200	SS 206 AR	+	Su 25 May	F 30 May	5	3	121	135	14	14€	70€	Camp Card No dep
4. Valence	Aix-en-Provence 0442261428	Camping Arc en Ciel 13100		+	F 30 May	W 18 June	19	4	125	130	15	21.7€	412.3€	0
5. Aix-en-Provence	Avignon 0490806350	Camping le Pont d'Avignon 84000	AR C Qual		W 18 June	Su 6 July	18	4	51	57	6	20.44	368.76	124.63€
6. Avignon	Montclar (Carcassonne 046826453	Domaine d'Arnauteille 11250	Yelloh village C Qual	+	Su 6 July	Th 10 July	4	4	137	164	18		166€	51€
7. Montclar	Lanne (Carcassonne 0562454005	Camping la Bergerie 65380 10amp	AR C Qual		Th 10 July	Su 13 July	3	3	147	164	14	16.9€	50.7€	0
8. Lanne	St Girons Plage 0558479014	Eurosol St Girons Plage 40560		+	Su 13 July	Su 27 July	14	4	76	115	8	37 32	513	125€
9. St Girons Plage	St Cyprien 0553291370	Domaine le Cro Magnon 24220	CC 73 SS 162	+	Su 27 July	Su 10 Aug	14	4	160	208	9		456.84€	107€
10. St Cyprien	Ingrandes 0549026147	Le Petit Trianon de St Ustre 86220 30 Euro	Cast 39 SS 145	+	Su 10 Aug	M 18 Aug	8	4	91	208	4	30.18€? 12.5 dep	241.44€+ 60.36€+	12.5 dep
11. Ingrandes	Saumur 0241512292 Varennes	L'Etang de la Breche 49730	Cast 23 SS 137	+ no dra	M 18 Aug	M 8 Sept	21	4	62	76	8		495.50€	133€
12. Saumur	Bernieres sur Mer 0231966709	Camping le Havre de Berniere 14990 10amp 20.70 Euro			M 8 Sept	Su 14 Sept	6	4	144	190	16	14€	84€	0 Camp Card
13. Bernieres sur Mer	Ferry	Ouistreham 14150			Su 14 Sept					10				

months off from work. It was lovely to see Simon Broomhall and to be able to thank him personally. He was also pleased to see me and asked for a copy of The One Show that I had featured in. He suggested that I should have a routine scan to check on what was going on inside so this was booked at Worcester.

Meanwhile, I was discharged from St Richard's but allowed to visit right up to the time I would be going away; this was completely fair. I had gained so much from going there and there were others waiting on the list.

22 *Frightened by Dr. Who*

It was in this relaxed but excited mood that we were all sitting around the television and watching an important episode of Dr Who. The story was gripping, but as I was sitting there I suddenly felt something which might be described as a bee sting or a sharp needle piercing the base of my neck on the right. This developed further to a feeling of the sting swelling or filling up into a ball and when I touched this point, I could feel a round lump the size of a pea which could be moved slightly when pressed. My throat also had a cutting feeling within.

I was worried but did not want to disturb the programme by something that could be nothing so I waited till it had finished. I then told Mark about the lump and said that I would feel happier if I phoned the out-of-hours doctor. This happened to be a female doctor who had suffered cancer herself; she told me that people who have cancer worry about any lump and she was sure this was nothing to be concerned about. If I had a sore throat, then the immune system would react and this would cause the lymph glands to swell. I felt reassured by this but the next day, my throat was getting worse. I was also sweating an awful lot and could not get comfortable; the blood was absolutely boiling inside me. I had made an appointment to see my GP about this as Dr. Farrago had said that I would be at no more risk than anyone else if I took

HRT treatment for menopausal symptoms. On seeing the sweat dripping off my hands, my GP put me on some HRT tablets and told me to double the dose if I needed to. She discussed my throat problem along with the fact that our trip was fast approaching and she took a swab of my throat to test for infection. When this turned out to be clear, I was still worried and so pleased that Mr Broomhall had booked me a scan which was to be carried out within the next couple of days. I told the radiologist about the lumps in my throat and he looked quite concerned. However, he could not find a vein big enough to insert the canula I needed in my arm for the contrast fluid; my veins had become rather faint with all the injections I had been given over time. Contrast fluid is passed into the vein during the scan to show up the details more clearly. Nonetheless, he did the scan without this and took particular note of my neck.

Time was passing quickly and the worry was growing; it was getting more and more difficult for me to talk with the soreness in my throat. I tried to contact Dr Farrago to make an urgent appointment but was unable to get a reply from my messages so I sought help from St Richard's. They were fantastic to me and I was able to see the doctor there who got the results of the scan for me. She went through the medical details and explained what it had said. There were several clusters of swollen lymph nodes around the aorta, mediastinum or chest and neck. She advised me to see Dr Farrago before any further planning was done. Mary, a nurse at the hospice, who has been such a support to me throughout, spoke to Dr Farrago's secretary; he was on annual leave at the time which was why I had a problem contacting him, but an appointment was made for me to see him that Tuesday, just a few days before our planned holiday.

Mark and I didn't know how to think; we couldn't look forward to the holiday but it could still be possible; there was a chance that this was just a reaction from the operation. I saw Dr Balimore on Tuesday; a lovely, understanding man. My CEA level had gone up to 7.2 and he could feel lumps on my throat and under my right arm.

'You need to have a biopsy,' he said and arranged for it to be done immediately. I was taken to the lower floor of the hospital and was seen almost immediately. The lady who did the analysis of the biopsy talked me through what was to happen and the consultant then came to take the biopsy. He held an instrument that looked like a small rechargeable drill, the type you can use without a plug. There was a fine needle fixed to this. It looked frightening but he assured me that it would hurt less than an injection; it just looked so awful. He was right. In fact, I was able to continue talking while he inserted the needle into the lump on my neck. He held it there a while and it made quite a noise as it syringed out some fluid and then he did the same again to take a second sample. I was treated really kindly and the analyst promised that the results would be sent to Dr Farrago the next day.

Again, I could not get in touch with Dr Farrago; he was such a busy man and attended meetings all over the country in addition to his busy schedule. It was Wednesday and my last proposed day at St Richard's. I had received no contact regarding the biopsy but Dr Susan got a copy of the scan report faxed to her at the hospice. I was taken to a side room; Mary came in with me and they told me the awful news so sensitively. The report stated that the lymph showed adeno carcinoma, the same cancer as my primary, so my cancer had spread. I was knocked back completely. Mary was so kind; she stayed with me and David, the chaplain, came in to sit with me till Mark arrived. I had to phone the news to Mark at work; poor Mark, having to cope with all this. Mary suggested that I wait at the hospice rather than go back to an empty house. What an awful disease this was; but we mustn't give up; we have to keep on fighting it. It was distressing to give Mum the news; we had all hoped that the cancer was cleared.

The next day, Thursday, Dr Farrago left his meeting to phone me and to say how sorry he was. He said that we could go away for two weeks if we wished and then start chemo treatment but I wanted to catch this thing as quickly as I could. I told him how difficult it was to talk and that it was getting worse by the day.

'When would you like to start the treatment?' he asked me.

I replied, 'Tomorrow!'

He told me that it would have to be Tuesday for his clinic which I knew. I would be put on a very strong dose of Irinotecan alone but he was straight in telling me that there was now only a ten percent success rate at this point. Well, there was still a chance, so I must go for it, however small.

After all the preparations, this was a major setback. We had done so much and all in vain. The Avastin had not worked post-operatively. I had been prepared to accept death a year ago but I was not prepared to accept it now; I just did not feel the same; it was really odd.

23 *Do I Still Believe in Miracles?*

It is a peculiar feeling to look forward to something that will actually knock you for six but I wanted treatment so badly; yes, it may only be a ten percent chance but it was a chance. The worst thing was to have to tell my sons the bad news; they had already been so strong. I decided that we would delay telling Aidan as he had his important third year exams in a couple of weeks; instead, we told him that I had to have some checks as there were some concerns so we would have to postpone the trip to France.

Mum came back down and she accompanied me to my chemo on the Tuesday along with Mark and she stayed with me for the whole day. The place was much busier now and there had been some changes but all the nurses came to talk to me when they had a moment and were as caring as always. The new course of irinotecan on its own had a dreadful effect on me. I could feel my cheeks and eyes twitching as it went in and that sweet chemical taste trickled through my throat; the memories of this drug were actually horrific and now the dose was stronger. By the end of the treatment I was dizzy as well and felt so weak when I started to walk. My speech was slurred as though I had been drinking. Mum had to steady me in the corridor and Mark supported me outside to the car. All the thoughts returned of sweating chemicals in bed, dryness in your eyes and mouth, sore feet and hands and loss of taste and of your memory. This is a peculiar reaction referred to as 'chemo brain' and suffered by many patients on these drugs.

I remember Delia at the hospice saying to me, 'Are you really prepared to go through all this again?'

'Yes, definitely,' was my response.

My hair started to fall much sooner this time and I was allowed another wig. Mark and I went off to Wills Wigs again and knew the routine this time. I had seen a lighter coloured, shorter styled streaked wig on their website and it had caught my eye so I asked to try that one. The lady in the shop was as helpful as ever and she brought even more similar styles for me to compare. Mark and I had some fun with him trying on some of the wigs before me when the lady was out of the room but she caught him at it and joined in with our silliness. Tracy shaved my head again for me at St Richard's and trimmed the wig as the fringe was quite long; she was great and it was quite comfortable with her as she was like a friend. People never gave up with you at St. Richard's as though it wasn't worth spending time on you; everyone was treated with respect and a future.

My new routine was now in place and we would go forwards from this point. At least my treatments would be every three weeks again which gave me a little time in-between to do something. What happened now was nothing but a miracle. As quickly as I had felt those lymph glands swelling and burning in my throat, I felt the easing of pain after treatment and within three days, I was able to talk comfortably again; you could hardly feel the lumps any more. On my second visit for treatment, Dr Farrago confirmed this and even the lumps under my arms had disappeared. The CEA level from my blood test confirmed that the chemo was working and the cancer was regressing. I was one of the lucky ten percent!

24 *Lazing on a Sunny Afternoon*

Gaining confidence in the situation, Mark and I decided to go to France after all; we planned this in June between the chemos. We would not go far but decided to go to an old favourite haunt near Cherbourg called 'Anse du Brick'. There is a beautiful campsite there, set up on a hillside overlooking a pretty bay, with a lighthouse and you can watch the sunset; quite a romantic setting of which Mark and I have fond memories. We planned a ten day stretch on our own in the caravan and booked a cottage on the site for Jevan and Aidan to join us for the final week, returning back to England with us. I was so looking forward to this as it really was quite special.

The proprietors remembered us and welcomed us happily; they allotted us a superb pitch not too far from the toilet block and we had running water and drainage to connect up to. The weather was gorgeous and to be in France again was bliss, having all the things we loved. We had been careful in checking up the nearest hospital that could treat cancer emergencies and Mark drove to the place to ensure we knew what to do. Again, I wrote down my treatment in French, should that be needed, and Dr Steel had given me antibiotics in case I caught any infection at all.

We thoroughly relaxed, met so many lovely people and enjoyed

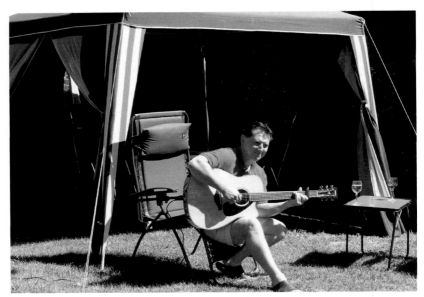

Lazing on a sunny afternoon!

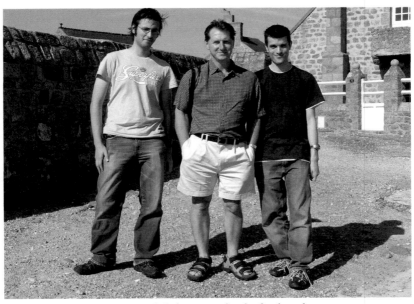

Jevan and Aidan came for the final week.

the sun. Even the ex-mayor of Nottingham and his wife came to sing with us one afternoon as Mark played his guitar. While I had a disability, it was always amazing to see other people coping with incredible situations far worse but so happily.

Jevan was allowed compassionate leave from work, which was lovely, and I can remember seeing him arrive with Aidan at the terminal in Cherbourg. It was many years since we had taken a holiday together and this was so special for me; I was overjoyed on seeing them and felt like a proud Mum.

25 *The PCT and Little Old Me*

Meanwhile, much was happening in the media; there was a great deal of interest as more people were coming forward and publicly stating how unfair the system was regarding access to these new drugs. Even less fair was the fact that each PCT seemed to have a different set of rules regarding funding the drugs; some people were given the drugs on the NHS whilst others were having to pay for all their treatment including scans. I was asked to discuss the matter with some people who were going through what I had already faced and I was pleased to hand over any information and help I had been given. The national newspapers were now taking an even greater interest and I was asked to give my details for case studies in The Guardian and The Sun with more photographers turning up and asking me to pose.

The Government now had to act as people were dying, having been refused all NHS treatment just because they had paid for one drug themselves. How was this different from dental treatment where you could go privately for some treatment and still have an NHS practitioner for other treatment? Professor Mike Richards was appointed to review the whole situation and report back to the House of Commons. There were debates on the radio and I was asked to do a recording for Radio 4 that would introduce one of these debates with the past president of the NHS and other people of high standing. It was all very nerve wracking but it was for a good cause and the BBC arranged and funded a taxi to the radio station for me. This recording was referred to in the House of Commons when Prof. Mike Richards presented his findings and it always seemed odd when people congratulated 'little old me' on something that seemed so natural to do. Mark and I were staying in Devon during the summer when the programme was broadcast and again, people on the caravan site at Kenford were stopping by to say how impressive it was. I was later phoned and offered £50 as a thank you for my part which was a pleasant surprise.

The summer was very wet but we made the most of it. I had forgotten what a beautiful place Devon was with its rolling hills and Mark and I enjoyed exploring on the coast and inland. However, the effects of the chemo were building up; I was so looking forward to my final, sixth treatment at the beginning of September and the scan that would hopefully bring good news. My CEA level had reduced to 1.6 which was the lowest it had ever been. It was absolutely wonderful to have all this confirmed and to be given a copy of the scan report which stated that the swelling in the lymph glands 'had totally regressed'. We were totally elated and always thanked Dr Farrago for his amazing expertise.

I would now be off chemo but I wanted to know what the expectations were.

'On average, the cancer returns in three months but it could be before or after that,' the doctor informed me. I now had it in my blood and it would return; the question was when. Pathologically, I had terminal cancer. I had a check-up arranged for a month away but was told that I must get back to him if I had any problems before that.

26 *Pictures at an Exhibition*

With no time to waste, Mark and I decided to take a final trip to France between now and the check-up in September and we chose to go to Honfleur, such a very pretty location, my favourite artist being Monet and our house filled with his prints; many of his paintings were created in the bay, now surrounded by beautiful little restaurants. We had visited the area about six years ago and loved it then; many of those memories flooded back and revisiting places now brought back happiness with a tinge of sadness from time to time. How lucky I was to be able to do all this, totally unexpected, now! We were certainly getting our fill of France and making up for some of what we couldn't do earlier, discovering places we had missed on previous visits, like the wealth and beauty of Deauville seafront.

While away, Ian Beaumont, from Bowel Cancer UK, phoned me and asked whether I would talk to the Sunday Telegraph. It was quite exciting to be photographed out there on a beautiful beach and buying the paper out there with the headline, 'For Barbara Moss the photographs of this summer's camping trip will be particularly special'. The family back at home were able to buy the paper and see us out there!

Other news came from Jevan who told us that he was planning

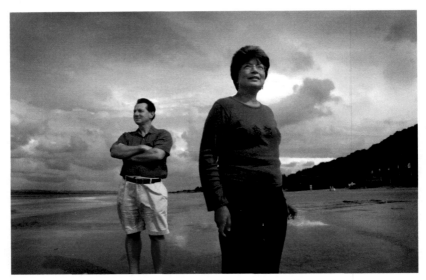

The photo in the Sunday Telegraph

to move into a flat with an old school friend, Dan, at the end of the month. I was happy at his excitement and progression though every Mum must feel a pang at this point, like the first time we left him on his own at Exeter University. We promised Jevan to give him the help he needed on our return and Mark kept to his word with finding, buying and moving heavy items up to his flat and feeling happy that he had been helped with a good start.

I wanted to share value time with Mark and equally with the family so we always tried to make arrangements for Jevan and Aidan to be home and for Mum to visit on our return from these trips. John and Eirian always invited us for their wonderful home cooked meals and entertained quite a crowd on numerous occasions.

Withdrawal symptoms and 'three months for the cancer to return' in the back of our minds, Mark and I booked the chalet at Anse du Brick again for two weeks in November.

27 *Oh My God!*

The 4th of November, 2008 was approaching, the date for the report from Prof. Mike Richards. Ian Beaumont had told me that we should expect some good news allowing the private purchase of drugs without the penalty of NHS treatment being withdrawn. What Prof. Richards actually recommended was far more than this and all his recommendations were accepted by the government. It was a wonderful feeling and many people thanked me for my contribution to this.

The government promised to review and give new guidelines to ensure all PCTs were uniform in their approach to these matters. They were also going to raise the amount they were prepared to spend on each person when they measured 'cost effectiveness' against life expectation and they were going to negotiate with the drug companies to lower their prices for a given length of time so that the NHS could afford them. Hence, as each drug was reviewed, more of the new drugs would be available to the average person on the NHS. It was fantastic to hear this and to think that a little person like me could help to make a difference to the nation. If you don't try, you can't hope.

With excitement, Friday the13th was fast approaching and our trip to Anse du Brick but thoughts were passing through my mind of asking for a refund of my costs. Would this even be considered retrospectively? Everything happens for a reason and one morning I had just decided to do some ironing so I switched on the radio, as I always do when I'm busy and on my own, and to my amazement, I heard one of the people I had tried to help previously talking on BBC Hereford and Worcester about this very topic. He had discussed the situation with the Chief Executive of Worcestershire PCT and had been told that he should not have had NHS treatment withdrawn. I wasted no time in contacting the PCT myself who said that they were reviewing our two cases but that they were the only two. I asked whether it would be helpful to send in all my hospital invoices and did this immediately. With no high hopes, I felt that there was nothing to lose, so it was worth a try.

Meanwhile, the internet is so useful for immediate updates and I read that three other people in London were asking for refunds. I pressed the PCT for a response, telling them that I was going to be away on the 13th. I had spoken to the chief accountant on the day before this and he promised me a letter on the morning of our departure. He told me that it was such a delicate matter, so it was being handled by their solicitor who had to word the letter; therefore, he preferred not to say anything himself. The post arrived on Friday but there was nothing. Dismayed, I phoned the accountant's secretary and she informed me that the letter was on the Chief Executive's desk awaiting a signature and it would be delivered by hand within the hour.

Imagine my total shock when it was presented to me personally by a charming, smiling lady and I was offered a refund of all my costs less the cost of the drug, Avastin. I had spent a total of £21,005 and was being offered £13, 658! I really couldn't believe what was happening.

My instant reaction was to phone Mum to give her the news and to promise her half of this; she couldn't believe it either. I then sent a joint email to family and close friends and phoned Worcester News who had followed my story and had given it coverage so many times. The health editor asked me how I felt about it.

'Ecstatic!' I replied.

I had barely placed the receiver down when the phone rang and BBC Hereford and Worcester were asking me for an interview for the news report. I couldn't spare the time as I had to get ready for the French trip; we were planning to leave at about 5pm and I still had to get my clothes packed. They pleaded but I resisted. Within moments, BBC TV was asking me to send some photos for their news coverage. Mark set the recorder to tape the news that evening as we would not be here to see it. I also had to write a reply of acceptance to the PCT to drop in at their office on the way to Poole for the ferry. That done, I had the radio station back onto me, saying that they would come to the house and it would only take ten minutes. Please! This time, I agreed but knew full well that one had to be prepared for these things as it took quite a lot out of you.

I did the recording without a hitch apart from the phone ringing in the middle of it. They asked me what I would spend the money on and, of course, I replied that I would repay my Mum and return the rest to where it came from. I was pleased with the outcome and very surprised to have the recording played on every news broadcast of every hour that day, stating that I was one of the first two in the country known to have been given a refund from the PCT. It was strange to hear this and I was pleased to be going away from all the publicity. It was only that evening, as Mark and I sat in a bar whiling away the time before the ferry, that the whole thing struck me. Unbelievable, only a small chance, but it happened!

28 *One Step at a Time*

This was a wonderful send-off and we thoroughly enjoyed our time. Again, we visited old haunts near Cherbourg but we also explored some new. We visited the museum at St Mere Eglise where, during the Second World War, the American soldier, John Steel survived because his parachute got caught up on the church steeple. He feigned death as he hung there for the entire day; hence he was

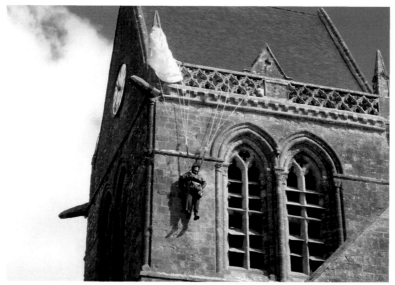

A replica of John Steel hanging from the steeple at St Mere Eglise

not shot down by the Germans. This was the setting for the film, 'The Longest Day'. There were photos of John Steel on his return to that site and it made you wonder what his thoughts must have been when he looked at that steeple around which life now goes on and the market thrives every Thursday because of his bravery. I remembered the time spent with Jevan and Aidan a few months back in Cherbourg and I always felt so lucky to have so much.

Time was passing so quickly and it was soon Christmas; there was not so much fuss about me any more which was a good thing and, for the first time, I was able to play a constructive part in preparing the meal for the day. Mum came over and on Sunday, we went to John and Eirian's which was special as Rachel, their eldest, had come over from New Zealand for a few days and we hadn't seen her for some years. We enjoyed a wonderful meal of lamb biryani and vegetable sambar, Eirian's speciality.

Into the New Year was such a strange feeling; 2009, what was I still doing here? Mark was being pressurised at work; he would not be able to have the same amount of time off, even though he had not been paid for any of it. I almost felt that I was being a nuisance by being alive but when I thought of my sons, that feeling soon went away. I still had a purpose and there was much to do. Aidan was in his last few months before his finals and Jevan was looking for work in IT. I also wanted to follow up what was happening after Prof. Mike Richards' review and planned to write to the Minister for Health, Alan Johnson. This was a low period that I had to pick myself out of and with the beautiful spring fast approaching, it didn't take long.

We spent a long stretch of time at home and Mark settled back to work; the depression did not seem to be hitting his company; on the contrary, there was a backlog of work to be done. I could see his predicament as, whilst he was good at his job, one of the best, he could not be in two places at once and he wanted to spend time with me. We have talked about this at length and have realised that our minds work quite differently; Mark looks at the picture as a whole while I see things in little bits. When the garden is full of weeds, I am happy to clear a small square of it; that way, I know it will be finished one day. Do nothing and you will never achieve your goal. This is how I have worked throughout my illness. When cooking, I would prepare the meat and vegetables first, then rest, returning later to actually do the cooking.

I feel that what we have always held on to strongly from the day of Dr. Hailer's news is our spirit of hope and it has got us so far. The last two years have given us so much that would seem impossible to achieve: my tumour shrinking sufficiently to enable resection; the swellings in my lymph receding completely when there was only a ten percent chance for this; the Government's U-turn on allowing private treatment alongside NHS care and my partial refund of costs for my chemotherapy. These have all been major events and I feel happy to have played some part in the change that will help others. One little step allowed the next to happen but it was always the first move which was the important one.

29 *Precious Moments*

This is my longest stretch without chemo and we have been told that the cancer will definitely return. In fact, when I asked Dr Farrago again,

'What are my chances now? I've lasted three months. Does that give me more hope for the next three?'

He answered, 'No. We just can't tell. You've already exceeded all expectation.'

I feel greedy to ask for more time because I've already been given so much. Sometimes, like yesterday, when I was weeding the garden, something I haven't been able to do for over two years, I almost feel 'normal'. It is lovely to be able to do normal things; things that other people may find a drudge. It would be lovely to just forget about the illness too but I feel that learning to live with cancer is the most important thing. While Dr Farrago's words rest in the back of my mind, I realise that having the illness has also given me precious moments that I would not otherwise have experienced and I hope that this gives me the strength for what lies ahead.

I still go to St Richard's on a Wednesday and have made many friends there, but two years on I can see that I am one of the only cancer suffering patients left from when I started going there. The chaplain has told me that there is something different about me; she feels that I have been blessed.

To return to where I started and to relive my journey makes me realise what others around me have been through on my account; I have truly been lucky. When the cancer does return, we will all be more prepared because we have had time to come to terms with the situation. I'm pleased to have been able to give you a brief insight into this journey but there is one person who understands all this more than anyone else: my teddy, Bobby, Mark's present to me on my first stay in hospital. He has always been there: at home, in hospital, on holiday, day and night. He's always peeping in my bed!

And every night, when Mark curls around me, holds me tight, and kisses me on the shoulder, I know that he's praying that I won't be taken from him.